Aromatherapy Oils

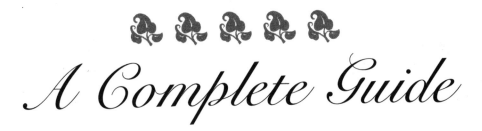

A Complete Guide

Carol Schiller &
David Schiller

Illustrated by Jeffrey Schiller

Library of Congress Cataloging-in-Publication Data

Schiller, Carol.
    Aromatherapy oils : a complete guide / by Carol Schiller
and David Schiller ; illustrated by Jeffrey Schiller.
        p.   cm.
    Includes index.
    ISBN 0-8069-6112-0
    1. Aromatherapy. I. Schiller, David, 1942–   . II. Title.
RM666.A68S354   1996
615'.321—dc20
                                                        96-24163
                                                        CIP

1 3 5 7 9 10 8 6 4 2

Published by Sterling Publishing Company, Inc.
387 Park Avenue South, New York, N.Y. 10016
© 1996 by Carol Schiller and David Schiller
Distributed in Canada by Sterling Publishing
c/o Canadian Manda Group, One Atlantic Avenue, Suite 105
Toronto, Ontario, Canada M6K 3E7
Distributed in Great Britain and Europe by Cassell PLC
Wellington House, 125 Strand, London WC2R 0BB, England
Distributed in Australia by Capricorn Link (Australia) Pty Ltd.
P.O. Box 6651, Baulkham Hills, Business Centre, NSW 2153, Australia
Manufactured in the United States of America
All rights reserved

Sterling ISBN 0-8069-6112-0

Acknowledgments

Many thanks to the special people who helped make this book possible:
Ken Tamblyn
Ray and Vanda Aka
Roslyn Blumenthal
Dave Weidinger
Susan Sherard
The staff and librarians at the Phoenix and Glendale Public Libraries in Arizona
and
The people at Sterling Publishing Company:
Sheila Anne Barry, Acquisitions Director
John Woodside, Editorial Director
Charles Nurnberg, Executive Vice President
Every writer knows the importance of having a good editor. We especially thank Hazel Chan, our editor,
for her professionalism and dedicated efforts, which contributed to improving the quality of *Aromatherapy Oils*
and made the editing process a pleasant experience.

Table of Contents

Aromas open the gateway of the mind and bring
forth memories, feelings, and emotions.
All of us are affected—some more so than others.
David Schiller

INTRODUCTION:

Aromatherapy Over the Years

Since the beginning of recorded history, aromatic plants have been used to scent, beautify, and heal the body. In ancient times, wealthy Egyptians luxuriated in the pleasures of bathing in scented waters, indulging in a delightful fragrant massage, and perfuming their bodies with enchanting oils and ointments. The priests were the first perfumers and healers to dispense aromatics by preparing blends for the kings, queens, and high dignitaries of temples and governments. During religious ceremonies, they used aromatic waters in the anointing rituals, and burned incense in an effort to protect against evil spirits and help the worshippers concentrate on their prayers. When the pharaohs died, their bodies were wrapped with fabric containing cinnamon, myrrh, cedarwood, and other resins and oils. This mummification method was confirmed to have been effective when modern-day archaeologists excavated the mummies and found them to be well preserved in their original burial chambers.

The ancient Romans lavishly perfumed their bodies and scented everything from military flags to the walls of their homes. Eventually, Rome became the bathing capital of the world with one thousand public bath houses located throughout the city for people to bathe, socialize, and afterwards enjoy a pampering massage with scented oils and unguents.

The art of extracting the volatile essences from plants was initiated by the Egyptians, who heated them in clay containers. Two centuries later, Greek alchemists invented the distillation process, which further developed the use of essences for religious and therapeutic purposes. By 1000 A.D., the Arabic physician, Avicenna, per-fected the extraction method by introducing the cooling system into the distillation process and, thereby, creating the most potent essences with stronger fragrances.

During the 14th century, the Great Plague devastated Europe and Asia, killing millions of people. All aromatic substances available were used for their antiseptic properties to fight off the dreaded disease. Cedar, clove, cypress, pine, sage, rosemary, and thyme were burned in the streets, hospitals, and sickrooms in a desperate attempt to prevent the spread of the epidemic. It was reported that perfumers and those who handled and used aromatics of various kinds were virtually immune to the ravages of the plague and survived.

The study of the therapeutic effectiveness of essential oils was further advanced by René-Maurice Gattefosse, a French cosmetic chemist. In the early 1920s, while working in his laboratory, Gattefosse accidentally burned his hand and immediately immersed it into the nearest cold liquid, which happened to have been a container of lavender oil. Surprisingly, the pain lessened and the reaction of redness, inflammation, and blistering was drastically reduced. In addition, the wound healed very quickly and no scar developed. After this incident, Gattefosse decided to dedicate the rest of his life to the study of the remarkable healing properties of the essential oils and coined the term "aromatherapy" in 1928.

Inspired by Gattefosse's work, Jean Valnet, a French medical doctor, exclusively used the essential oils to treat the battle wounds of the French soldiers during World War II. Dr. Valnet's extensive use of essences gained him official recognition in France and acknowledged aromatherapy as a true therapy. His book, *The Practice of Aromatherapy*, is a classic publication on the subject.

About the same time as Dr. Valnet was practicing aromatherapy, Madame Marguerite Maury, a biochemist, pursued her study of the cosmetic and therapeutic uses of the essential oils, and was later awarded the Prix International for her work in natural skin care.

Today, the use of essential oils by people worldwide is steadily becoming more widespread as greater numbers of individuals become aware of the myriad life-enhancing properties of these remarkable substances. These precious essences help balance and put us in greater harmony with the natural world. They protect us with their antibacterial properties, reduce our stress, and give us comfort, reassurance, and pleasure.

Some of the oils can produce instantaneous results that are easily recognizable, while others perform their work at a slower pace in a relatively unnoticeable subtle way. Only those people who use the oils on a regular basis can begin to understand and fully appreciate and respect their miraculous value.

Aromatherapy offers us a chance to reach out to our forgotten past. By looking to nature with all its benefits and beauty, we can take advantage of the valuable wisdom of the ages from our ancestors and benefit from this very precious gift of aromatic essential oils.

CHAPTER 1

Safety, Handling, and Selection of Oils

Essential oils can be extremely beneficial when used properly; therefore, please follow these guidelines:

- Essential oils are highly concentrated substances and should be diluted in a carrier oil such as sweet almond oil before applying on the skin in order to prevent skin irritation. (*For proper blending see Chapter 2.*) If any skin irritation should occur as a result of the essential oils, immediately apply additional carrier oil or lavender oil to the area. This will quickly soothe the skin.

- When applying essential oils on the skin, using a spray mist, or taking a scented bath, be careful not to get the oils into the eyes.

- Care must be taken when using carrier and essential oils during pregnancy. Many of the oils have a stimulating effect on the uterus, which can be very helpful at the appropriate time to facilitate childbirth. However, if those oils are used prior to the time of childbirth, they can bring on premature labor. Even certain common foods, spices, and vegetable oils, such as celery, carrots, parsley, basil, bay leaves, marjoram, and safflower oil, can stimulate uterine contractions.

- Small amounts (2–3 drops at one time) of the following essential oils are safe during pregnancy: Bergamot, Cananga, Coriander, Cypress, Frankincense, Geranium, Ginger, Grapefruit, Lavandin, Lavender, Lemon, Lime, Mandarin, Neroli, Orange, Patchouli, Petitgrain, Sandalwood, Spearmint, Tangelo, Tangerine, Tea Tree, Temple Orange, Ylang-Ylang. Sesame oil can be used as a carrier oil.

- A woman nursing her baby should exercise caution when using the essential oils, since the effects of the oils will be readily passed on to the infant.

- If a person is highly allergic, a simple test can determine if there is any sensitivity to a particular oil. Rub a drop of carrier oil on the upper chest area, and in 12 hours, check if there is redness or any other skin reaction. If the skin is clear, place 1 drop of an essential oil, diluted in 20 drops of the same carrier oil, and again rub on the upper chest area. If there is no skin reaction after 12 hours, both carrier and essential oil can be used.

- Do not consume alcohol, except a small glass of wine with a meal, in the time period when using essential oils.

- Do not use the essential oils while on medication; the oils might interfere with the medicine.

- The following oils can be especially irritating to the skin and must be used with extra care, particularly by those with dry skin: Ajowan, Allspice, Anise, Anise (*Star*), Basil, Bay (*West Indian*), Bay (*Sweet*), Bergamot, Benzoin, Birch (*Sweet*), Cinnamon (*Bark and Leaf*), Citronella, Clove, Cornmint, Cumin, Elecampane, Fennel, Ginger, Gingergrass, Grapefruit, Lemon, Lemon Verbena, Lemongrass, Lime, Litsea Cubeba, Mandarin, Massoia Bark, Melissa, Orange, Oregano, Pepper (*Black*), Parsley, Peppermint, Peru Balsam, Pine, Savory, Spearmint, Tagetes, Tangelo, Tangerine, Temple Orange, Thyme, Wintergreen.

- After an essential oil blend is applied on the skin, avoid for at least 4 hours sunbathing, sauna/steam room, aor a hot bath in order to prevent the possibility of skin irritation. This precaution is especially important when using citrus, phototoxic, and other essential oils that can irritate the skin.

- There are people with extremely sensitive skin who cannot tolerate the essential oils without having skin irritation. If this is the case, please discontinue use.

- When spilled on furniture, many essential oils will remove the finish; therefore, be careful when handling the bottles.

- Light and oxygen cause oils to deteriorate rapidly. Refrigeration does not prevent spoilage but diminishes the speed at which it occurs. Therefore, oils should be stored in brown-colored glass bottles in a dark and cool place.

- Always use a glass dropper when measuring drops of essential oil.

- Keep all bottles tightly closed to prevent the oils from evaporating and oxidizing.

- Always store essential oils out of sight and reach from children.

Methods of Extraction

The extraction process is a factor in determining the purity of the oil. Before purchasing carrier and essential oils, it is important to become knowledgeable of these methods.

Steam Distillation
Steam from boiling water is used to extract the essential oils from the plant material. The steam is then cooled and condensed into a liquid from which the oil is separated as it floats on top of the water. This method produces a good quality essential oil.

Carbon Dioxide Gas Extraction
Expensive high-technology equipment is used to extract the essential oils. It employs carbon dioxide gas (CO_2), high pressure, and low tempera-ture. This process produces an oil that retains a greater amount of aromatic components than by steam distillation. The scent of CO_2 extracted oil is more identical to that of the original plant.

Cold, Expeller, or Mechanically Pressed
Seeds, nuts, fruits, and vegetables are pressed without the use of heat; however, a large percent-age of these oils is usually refined afterwards using high heat and harsh chemicals.

Maceration
Flowers are soaked in hot oil until their cells rup-ture and the oil absorbs the essence.

Solvent Extraction
Solvents, such as hexane and other toxic chemi-cals, are used to extract the oil from the plant material. This method is less costly and more efficient in producing a greater amount of oil. However, toxic residues are left from the hexane, making it undesirable for those wanting pure oils. Absolute flower oils and a high percentage of commercial vegetable oils are extracted using this method.

Refining Process for Vegetal/Carrier Oils
After the oil has been extracted from the plant material, it is usually put through a refining process that includes these steps:

Degumming: Removes chlorophyll, vitamins, and minerals from the oil.

Refining: An alkaline solution called lye is added to refine the oil.

Bleaching: Fuller's earth is added as a bleaching agent and then filtered out, further removing nutritive substances. The oil at this stage becomes clear.

Deodorizing: The oil is deodorized by steam dis-tillation at high temperatures over 450°F (232°C) for 30–60 minutes.

Winterizing: The oil is then cooled and filtered. This process prevents the oil from becoming cloudy during cold temperatures. The finished product is nutrient deficient with only fatty acids remaining.

Selection of Quality Oils

It is unfortunate, but a high percentage of oils that are commonly sold to the public are adulterated. This is done in order to increase profits without much concern for the consequences to the consumers. Some of the adulteration can be comprised of adding a cheaper oil to a more expensive oil in order to "stretch" it. Many other more serious adulterations take place by adding synthetic as well as fractionalized components, which contaminate the oils. This practice is common knowledge in the essential oil industry and referred to as "making a soup." Each time the oil changes hands, the possibility increases for the original oil to become more diluted.

A few common examples of adulteration

Essential Oil	Adulterated with
Lavender	Lavandin
Neroli	Petitgrain
Pimento berry	Clove
Rose	Palmarosa
Rosemary	Eucalyptus
Patchouli	Gurjun Balsam
Peppermint	Cornmint
Sandalwood	Amyris
Ylang-Ylang	Cananga

Synthetic oils and oils that are extracted by chemical or petroleum solvents should never be used. The man-made chemicals that replicate the aromas of natural oils do not contain the beneficial properties of the pure plant oils. As a matter of fact, many of these synthetic compounds can be very irritating to the nervous system and entire body. The oils that are solvent-extracted contain toxic residues from the solvent and can be harmful as well.

The highest-grade and most effective oils are produced from plants that are grown wild and away from polluted sources, or are cultivated by natural farming methods without the use of pesticides, herbicides, or any other unnatural substances. It is important to select for purchase unrefined carrier oils that are cold, expeller, or mechanically pressed, and essential oils that have been either CO_2 extracted, steam distilled, or, in the case of citrus fruit oils, cold pressed.

CHAPTER 2

Vegetal Oils and Butters

The following vegetal oils and butters are covered in this chapter:

Almond (*Sweet*)	Coconut**	Peanut
Apricot Kernel	Corn	Pecan
Avocado*	Cottonseed	Pine Nut
Babassu	Evening Primrose*	Pistachio Nut
Beechnut	Flaxseed	Pumpkinseed*
Ben	Grapeseed	Rice Bran
Black Currant Seed*	Hazelnut	Rose Hip Seed
Borage*	Jojoba*	Safflower
Brazil Nut	Kiwifruit Seed	Sea Buckthorn
Calophyllum	Kukui Nut	Sesame
Camellia	Macadamia Nut	Shea Butter**
Canola (*Rapeseed*)	Mango*	Sisymbrium*
Carrot Root*	Mangosteen (*Kokum Butter*)	Soybean*
Carrot Seed	Neem	Sunflower
Cashew Nut*	Olive	Walnut
Castor	Palm**	Wheat Germ*
Chaulmoogra	Palm Kernel	
Cocoa Butter**	Passion Fruit Seed	

Vegetal oils are derived from seeds, nuts, fruits, and vegetables. Many of these oils are used as a carrier oil to dilute essential oils so that the blend can be applied safely on the skin.

The vegetal/carrier oils denoted with one asterisk (*) can be combined into one of the other vegetal/carrier oils so that they comprise a percentage of the total mixture. This is usually done to help create a blend that has a smooth texture and can be easily absorbed into the skin during a massage.

The specific percentage is indicated under the "Practical Uses" listed in this chapter for each individual oil. For example, a good formula for 1 ounce (30 ml) of a skin-rejuvenating facial oil would be:

Borage*	1 teaspoon—(17%)
Pine Nut	5 teaspoons—(83%)

When combining essential oils with the carrier oil, blend 12 to 30 drops of the essential oils into 1 ounce (30 ml) of the carrier oil.

Thus, with the addition of the essential oils, the formula for the skin-rejuvenating facial oil becomes:

Pine Nut	3 teaspoons
Sisymbrium	2 teaspoons
Borage*	1 teaspoon
Sandalwood	8 drops
Bois de Rose	7 drops
Patchouli	5 drops

An example of two massage oil blends for relax-ation/stress reduction would be:

Almond (*Sweet*)	4 teaspoons
Mandarin	5 drops
Lemongrass	5 drops
Lavender	5 drops
Ylang-Ylang	5 drops

✦ ✦ ✦

Evening Primrose*	1 teaspoon
Hazelnut	5 teaspoons
Litsea Cubeba	8 drops
Sandalwood	8 drops
Chamomile (*Roman*)	5 drops
Vetiver	5 drops
Bergamot	4 drops

The vegetal/carrier oil denoted with two asterisks (**) hardens at room temperature and is appro-priate as an ingredient when making an ointment.

Helpful Measurements

2 tablespoons	= 1 ounce
6 teaspoons	= 1 ounce
1 teaspoon	= 5 ml
1 tablespoon	= 15 ml
1 ounce	= 30 ml
1 teaspoon	= 100 drops
1 tablespoon	= 300 drops

PLEASE NOTE: Practical Uses refers to tried and proven everyday aromatherapy uses. Documented Properties refers to properties documented in other publications.

ALMOND (Sweet)

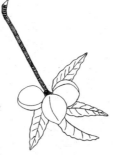

Botanical Name: *Prunus amygdalus, P. dulcis*
Family: *Rosaceae*

The oil is obtained from the nut of the tree.

History and Information

- Sweet almond is native to Asia and the Mediterranean region. The medium-sized tree grows to a height of about 35 feet, has pinkish-white flowers, and belongs to the rose family.

There are approximately fifty species of the wild almond trees but only a few varieties pro-duce a sweet kernel. The cultivated types of almond trees require cross-pollination with another variety.

- Pliny, the Roman herbalist, listed the use of almonds as a treatment for many disorders.

- Throughout the years, women used almond oil on their face to give it a nice complexion.

- In Ayurvedic medicine, almonds are said to improve the eyesight. The seed and oil are con-sidered aphrodisiacs.

- In Europe, before the 18th century, almonds were powdered, soaked in water, and made into a nutritional beverage as a substitute for milk.

- In China, almonds and brown rice are ground up into a powder and mixed with water and honey to help or prevent dry throats and other dry conditions.

- Almonds are rich in calcium, potassium, mag-nesium, iron, and phosphorus, and have an oil content of 54%. Almost all almonds grown in the United States are produced in California, which supplies more than half of the world's population. The second largest producer of nuts is Spain. Almonds do poorly in tropical regions since high humidity during ripening may cause rancidity to develop in the kernels. Almonds are the most consumed of all the nuts.

Practical Uses

Skin care; moisturizing
Suntanning oil
The carrier/base oil is used to dilute essential oils in aromatherapy for massage oils and other for-mulations.

Documented Properties

Alterative, Anti-inflammatory, Antilithic, Antipruritic, Astringent, Carminative, Demul-cent, Diuretic, Emollient, Galactagogue, Laxative, Nervine, Tonic, Vulnerary

APRICOT KERNEL

Botanical Name: *Armeniaca vulgaris, Prunus armeniaca*
Family: *Rosaceae*

The oil is obtained from the kernel of the fruit.

History and Information

- Apricot is native to Asia. The tree grows to a height of about 35 feet , and has white to pink flowers and an orange-yellow fruit.

- The Hunza women use the oil to maintain a nice complexion and wrinkle-free skin.

- In northern China, the apricot tree is primarily cultivated for its edible nuts, which are almost identical to almonds.

- The oil is similar in texture and properties to almond oil.

Practical Uses

Skin care; moisturizing
The carrier/base oil is used to dilute essential oils in aromatherapy for massage oils and other formulations.

Documented Properties

Antitussive, Nourishing (*Skin*)

AVOCADO

Botanical Name: *Persea americana, Persea gratissima*
Family: *Lauraceae*

The oil is obtained from the kernel and fruit of the tree.

History and Information

- Avocado is an evergreen tree native to the Americas. The tree grows to a height of about 30–60 feet, and has dark green oval leaves and greenish-yellow flowers that develop into a yellow, green, red, or purple-colored fruit. The pulp is soft and buttery with a large kernel inside. Avocado grows in many tropical regions.

- Avocados were highly esteemed by the Aztec and Maya Indians.

- The unripe fruit is poisonous. Its powdered seed mixed with cheese is used to poison mice.

- In the country of Zaire, a beer is brewed from the avocado leaves.

- Avocado oil is very nourishing to the skin and known to contain vitamins A and E, and especially large amounts of vitamin D and potassium. The avocado has the highest protein content of any fruit. The oil is extensively used in cosmetics.

Practical Uses

Skin care; moisturizing; purifies the skin
The carrier/base oil is used to dilute essential oils in aromatherapy for massage oils and other formulations. For massage oils, it is best to mix 20% of the avocado oil with another carrier oil before adding the essential oils.

Documented Properties

Hepatic, Rejuvenator, Restorative (*Skin*), Tonic, Vulnerary

COMMENTS: Poisoning of animals feeding on the leaves, bark, and fruit of the avocado tree has been reported. However, the ripe fruit and oil, in moderate amounts, seem safe to humans.

BABASSU

Botanical Name: *Orbignya barbosiana*
Family: *Arecaceae*

The oil is derived from the kernels of the fruit.

History and Information

- Babassu is a wild and fast-growing palm tree in Brazil that reaches a height of about 66 feet. The fruits are fleshy with a hard shell on the outside. Babassu tastes and smells like coconut but yields a higher amount of oil. The tree is also known as aguassu or babacu.

- The Amazonian people use every part of the tree for food, shelter, utensils, and clothing.

- The properties of the oil are similar to, and sometimes substituted for, coconut oil. Babassu oil is used in cooking, margarine, fuel, lubricants, detergents, soaps, and cosmetics. The oil does not turn rancid as quickly as the other palm tree oils.

Practical Uses

Skin care; soothing; helps with stretch marks
The carrier/base oil is used to dilute essential oils in aromatherapy for massage oils and other formulations.

Documented Properties

Anthelmintic, Antibacterial, Antidote, Antiseptic, Aperient, Aphrodisiac, Astringent, Depurative, Diuretic, Hemostatic, Laxative, Purgative, Refrigerant, Stomachic, Vermifuge

BEECHNUT

Botanical Name: *Fagus grandifolia, F. sylvatica*
Family: *Fagaceae*

The oil is derived from the nuts of the tree.

History and Information

- Beechnut is a deciduous tree native to the northern hemisphere. The tree grows to a height of about 80–150 feet. The nuts are enclosed in prickly burs. In the fall season, they open as the nuts mature. There are ten species of the beechnut tree.

- Pliny, the Roman herbalist, praised the nuts as a food.

- North American Indians also valued the beechnuts as a food.

- In France, ground beechnuts have been made into a drink as a substitute for coffee.

- The nuts contain a high protein content of about 20% and yield an oil content of about 50%. The oil is used as a salad oil or a substitute for butter. The nuts can be eaten fresh, dried, or roasted, but the fresh nuts spoil in a relatively short period of time.

- The wood of the tree is strong and hard, and used for furniture.

Practical Uses

Skin care; soothing

BEN

Botanical Name: *Moringa oleifera, M. pterygosperma*
Family: *Moringaceae*

The oil is derived from the seeds of the tree.

History and Information

- Ben is a deciduous tree native to Asia and Africa. The tree grows to a height of about 35 feet, and has leathery leaves, white or yellow fragrant flowers, and long pods containing seeds. Ben is also known as the drumstick tree, horseradish tree, and benzolive tree.

- In folk medicine, the oil was used for skin problems.

- In Ayurvedic medicine, the leaves are used to relieve congestion and act as a poultice for injuries and swellings. The flowers are used as an aphrodisiac; the oil is used for gout and painful joints.

- The roots are fleshy and smell like horseradish. The fruit, leaves, and flowers are edible. The seeds yield approximately 40% oil and are used in salads, foods, artist paints, lubricants, soaps, cosmetics, and perfumery. The oil is scentless, colorless, and tasteless; it is resistant to oxidation and has a high melting point.

Practical Uses

Skin care

Documented Properties

Antibacterial, Antidote, Cholagogue, Depurative, Diuretic, Emetic, Estrogenic, Expectorant, Galactagogue, Purgative, Rubefacient, Stimulant, Tonic, Vermifuge

BLACK CURRANT SEED

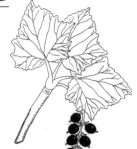

Botanical Name: *Ribes nigrum*
Family: *Grossulariaceae*

The oil is obtained from the seeds of the plant.

History and Information

- Black currant is a deciduous plant native to Europe and Asia. The plant grows to a height of about 7 feet, and has greenish flowers and edible black berries.

- Black currants have been cultivated since the beginning of the 18th century. They were considered a remarkable life-prolonging food; the leaves were used as a tea.

- Black currant buds produce an essential oil that is an ingredient in expensive perfumes; the berries are made into jam, syrup, and liqueurs.

- Black currants are one of the richest sources of vitamin C.

Practical Uses

Helps premenstrual stress
Relieves menstrual pain; reduces inflammation
Skin care; soothing; healing
The carrier/base oil is used to dilute essential oils in aromatherapy for massage oils and other formulations. For massage oils, it is best to mix 20% of black currant seed oil with another carrier oil before adding the essential oils.

Documented Properties

Antibacterial, Antidiarrhoeic, Antilithic, Antirheumatic, Antisclerotic, Antiscorbutic, Diaphoretic, Diuretic, Hepatic

BORAGE

Botanical Name: *Borago officinalis*
Family: *Boraginaceae*

The oil is obtained from the seeds of the plant.

History and Information

- Borage is native to the Mediterranean region. The plant grows to a height of about 2–4 feet, and has star-shaped, sky-blue colored flowers and large pointed oval leaves. The scent of the plant is similar to a cucumber.

- The ancient Celtic warriors drank a wine made with borage before battle to increase their courage.

- Pliny, the Roman herbalist, and Dioscorides, the Greek physician, recommended borage for lifting one's spirits.

- In France, borage is used as a febrifuge and for pulmonary discomforts.

- The oil contains one of the highest amounts of gamma-linoleic acid (GLA), which is said to help slow down the skin's aging process.

Practical Uses

Calming
Helps premenstrual stress
Relieves menstrual pain; reduces inflammation
Skin care; inflamed skin
The carrier/base oil is used to dilute essential oils in aromatherapy for massage oils and other formulations. For massage oils, it is best to mix 20% of borage oil with another carrier oil before adding the essential oils.

Documented Properties

Antidepressant, Antidote, Anti-inflammatory, Antirheumatic, Aperient, Astringent, Calmative, Decongestant, Demulcent, Depurative, Diaphoretic, Diuretic, Emollient, Expectorant (*Mild*), Febrifuge, Galactagogue, Hepatic, Hypotensor, Nervine, Refrigerant, Regenerator (*Skin*), Regulator (*Menstrual*), Sedative, Stimulant (*Mild*) (*Bowels*), Sudorific, Tonic

BRAZIL NUT

Botanical Name: *Bertholletia excelsa*
Family: *Lecythidaceae*

The oil is derived from the nuts of the tree.

History and Information

- The brazil nut is an evergreen tree grown in the Amazon forests of South America. The tree reaches a height of about 150 feet, and has white or yellow flowers. The casing for the nuts contains up to approximately twenty nuts and takes over a year to ripen on the tree.

- Brazil nuts tend to become rancid quickly unless they are stored in a closed container in a dry, dark, and cool place. The nut is also known as para nut, cream nut, and castanas nut.

Practical Uses

Skin care; moisturizing, soothing
The carrier/base oil is used to dilute essential oils in aromatherapy for massage oils and other formulations.

CALOPHYLLUM

Botanical Name: *Calophyllum inophyllum*
Family: *Guttiferae*

The oil is obtained from the kernel of the fruit.

History and Information

- Calophyllum is commonly found in tropical Asia. The tree grows to a height of about 10 feet and has flowers that emit a sweet fragrance. The flowers develop into clustered fruits that have a thin pulp and taste similar to an apple.

- The ancient Polynesians considered the calophyllum tree sacred because of its valuable medicinal properties. Calophyllum is still currently used by hospitals in Tahiti and surrounding areas.

- The Calophyllum kernels are dried in the sun and yield approximately 75% oil. The oil has a thick consistency similar to olive oil; it is also known as pinnay, dillo, domba, foraha, or tamanu oil.

Practical Uses

Skin care; healing to the skin
The carrier/base oil is used to dilute essential oils in aromatherapy for massage oils and other formulations.

Documented Properties

Analgesic, Anti-inflammatory, Regenerator (*Skin*)

CAMELLIA

Botanical Name: *Camellia japonica*
Family: *Theaceae*

The oil is obtained from the seeds of the plant.

History and Information

- Camellia grows wild in the mountains of Japan and China. The plant reaches a height of about 6–20 feet and has showy flowers that develop into seeds. Camellia belongs to a family of eighty species of evergreen trees and shrubs in Asia, and is a relative of the trees that produce tea leaves. The plant thrives in the colder climates of Asia, blossoming in the winter and even during snow.

- The oil has been used for centuries by Japanese women for skin and hair care.

- Camellia oil is also known as tsubaki oil; it is used in skin care products, as a seasoning for salads, and for cooking and frying.

- The oil oxidizes rapidly when exposed to air.

Practical Uses

Skin care; soothing
Hair care
The carrier/base oil is used to dilute essential oils in aromatherapy for massage oils and other formulations.

CANOLA (Rapeseed)

Botanical Name: *Brassica napus*
Family: *Brassicaceae*

The oil is obtained from the seeds of the plant.

History and Information

- The rape plant belongs to the same family as cabbage, and is also known as cole or coleseed.

The plant grows to a height of about 3 feet and has rows of yellow flowers.

- In Indonesia, the roots of the plant are used for sore throats and coughs.

Practical Uses

The carrier/base oil is used to dilute essential oils in aromatherapy for massage oils and other formulations.

COMMENTS: The original rape seeds contained 40% erucic acid, which is known to be harmful to the thyroid, kidneys, heart, and adrenals. The new genetically-altered plant variety now contains 1% of the toxic substance.

CARROT ROOT & CARROT SEED

Botanical Name: *Daucus carota*
Family: *Apiaceae*

Carrot root oil is obtained from the root of the plant. Carrot seed oil is obtained from the seeds.

History and Information

- Carrots are native to Afghanistan and the Mediterranean region. The plant grows to a height of about 1 foot and has white flower heads. Carrots are widely cultivated for food.

- Carrots were used in medicinal remedies during Roman and Grecian times, and only became recognized as an important food in the 16th century.

- Carrots help bring on menstruation and stimulate lactation; the seeds are used to eliminate intestinal worms.

- The oil is very high in beta carotene and vitamin A.

- Carrot root oil is used as a yellow food coloring and sunscreen in tanning lotions.

Practical Uses

Skin care; moisturizing
Brittle and dry hair
The carrier/base oil of carrot root is used to dilute essential oils in aromatherapy for massage oils and other formulations. For massage oils, it is best to mix 20% of carrot root oil with another carrier oil before adding the essential oils.

Documented Properties

Anthelmintic, Antilithic, Antipruritic, Antisclerotic, Aperitive, Astringent, Carminative, Diuretic, Emmenagogue, Galactagogue, Hemostatic, Hepatic, Laxative, Parasiticide, Rejuvenator (*Skin Cells*), Stimulant (*Uterine*), Tonic, Vasodilator, Vermifuge, Vulnerary

COMMENTS: Carrot seed is an essential oil.

CASHEW NUT

Botanical Name: *Anacardium occidentale*
Family: *Anacardiaceae*

The oil is derived from the nut of the tree.

History and Information

- Cashew nut is an evergreen tree native to tropical areas of Latin America. The tree grows to a height of about 40 feet and has pink flowers that develop into edible fruits known as cashew apples. The tree also produces a resin called cardol. Cashew belongs to the same family as the poison ivy, poison oak, poison sumac, mango, and pistachio.

- In Ayurvedic texts dating back to the 16th century, cashews were mentioned as a skin rejuvenator and appetizer.

- Throughout the years, in Latin America the leaves were applied on the skin to soothe burns, and the bark was made into tea and taken to relieve congestion.

- In Asia, the young shoots, leaves, and buds are eaten raw.

- India is the largest grower of cashew nuts.

- Cashew nuts are roasted in oil before being sold commercially.

- The nuts yield approximately 45% oil. The shell of the nut also yields an oil that is used as an insecticide.

Practical Uses

Skin care
The carrier/base oil is used to dilute essential oils in aromatherapy for massage oils and other formulations. For massage oils, it is best to mix 20% of cashew nut oil with another carrier oil.

Documented Properties

Aperitif, Rejuvenator (*Skin*)

CASTOR

Botanical Name: *Ricinus communis*
Family: *Euphorbiaceae*

The oil is obtained from the bean of the plant.

History and Information

- Castor is native to India. The plant grows to a height of about 5–12 feet, and has clusters of yellow or red flowers.

- The castor beans contain ricin, which is a deadly toxin. The ingestion of one to five seeds can be fatal to a child. In order to extract a ricin-free oil, the beans must be hulled and crushed at temperatures below 100°F. After the oil is extracted from the seeds, the ricin remains in the seed cake.

- Castor was one of the first medicinal plants known to humans. The beans were found in an ancient Egyptian tomb.

- The Egyptians added castor oil to beer and drank it as a purgative for cleansing their system.

- The oil has been applied on the breasts of nursing mothers to increase milk, relieve inflammation, soften the mammary glands, and as a lactagogue. It has also been used externally for abscesses, itching, dandruff, and hemorrhoids.

- The oil has a long shelf-life and is added to many food products.

Practical Uses

Blackheads
Hair and scalp care; dandruff

Documented Properties

Analgesic (*Hot Packs for Pain and Inflammation, recommended by Edgar Cayce*), Anti-inflammatory, Galactagogue, Laxative, Vermifuge (*Tapeworms*)

CHAULMOOGRA

Botanical Name: *Hypnocarpus kurzii, H. laurifolia, Oncoba echinata, Taraktagenos kurzii*
Family: *Flacourtiaceae*

The oil is derived from the seeds of the tree.

History and Information

- Chaulmoogra is an evergreen tree native to Asia. The tree grows to a height of about 50 feet, and has greenish flowers and leaves that can extend up to 10 inches long. There are forty varieties of chaulmoogra trees. The *Oncoba echinata* variety is known as the gorli shrub.

- Chaulmoogra oil has been used in Hindu medicine for many centuries for skin problems, leprosy, and muscle and joint ailments.

- Chaulmoogra nuts are popular in Asia.

Practical Uses

Skin care

Documented Properties

Analgesic, Restorative (*Skin*)

COMMENTS: The botanical species of *Hypnocarpus laurifolia* is safer to use than the other varieties of chaulmoogra, which have been found to be toxic.

COCOA BUTTER

Botanical Name: *Theobroma cacao*
Family: *Sterculiaceae*

The butter is obtained from the beans of the tree.

History and Information

- Cocoa is an evergreen tree native to Central America. The tree grows to a height of about 24 feet, and has large glossy leaves and small yellow flowers that develop into yellow or red fruits. The tree thrives along riverbanks.

- Cocoa was first introduced to Europe by Christopher Columbus, who learned of its use from the Aztecs.

- In South America, miners were given cocoa leaves to chew to increase their energy level and enable them to work long hours. Today, the leaves are used as a heart tonic.

- The beans are used in products such as skin lotions, creams, lipsticks, soaps, suppositories, and in the manufacturing of chocolate. An essential oil known as theobroma oil is produced from the fruit and beans of the tree.

- Theobromine is an alkaloid component of the cocoa bean, which is responsible for its stimulating effect.

Practical Uses

Stimulant
Skin and hair moisturizer

Documented Properties

Diuretic, Emollient, Moisturizer, Stimulant

COCONUT

Botanical Name: *Cocos nucifera*
Family: *Arecaceae*

The oil is obtained from the nut of the tree.

History and Information

- Coconut is a large evergreen palm found growing along the seashore in the tropics. The coconut tree reaches a height of about 100 feet and has small sweet-scented flowers. The tree is indispensable to the survival of millions of people, who rely on it as a primary source of food, drink, clothing, and shelter. The coconut fruit is regarded as one of the most important foods to one-third of the world's population.

- In Latin America, nursing mothers rub coconut milk on their breasts to reduce inflammation.

- Coconut has an oil content of 35%. It is used in foods, and in body care and industrial products.

Practical Uses

Skin care; soothing; helps with stretch marks
The carrier/base oil is used to dilute essential oils in aromatherapy for massage oils and other formulations. Coconut oil is generally solid at room temperature and, therefore, useful to make ointments.

Documented Properties

Anthelmintic, Antibacterial, Antidote, Antiseptic, Aperient, Aphrodisiac, Astringent, Depurative, Diuretic, Hemostatic, Laxative, Purgative, Refrigerant, Stomachic, Vermifuge

CORN

Botanical Name: *Zea mays*
Family: *Poaceae*

The oil is obtained from the kernels of the plant.

History and Information

- Corn is native to the Americas and belongs to the grass family. The plant can reach a height of up to 18 feet. The vegetable is a very important food staple to many people around the world.

- Corn was first cultivated in Mexico around 3400 B.C.

- The ground-up corncob and silk are used in China to relieve water retention and urinary stones.

- Corn only has an oil content of 4%; therefore, most of the oil produced is extracted through the use of toxic solvents and high temperatures.

- The color of the unrefined oil is dark gold with a popcorn scent. It is high in unsaturated fatty acids.

Practical Uses

Skin care; moisturizing, soothing

The carrier/base oil is used to dilute essential oils in aromatherapy for massage oils and other formulations.

Documented Properties

Diuretic, Tonic, Vulnerary

COTTONSEED

Botanical Name: *Gossypium species*
Family: *Malvaceae*

The oil is obtained from the seeds of the plant.

History and Information

- There are many different varieties of cotton plants cultivated throughout the world. The plant grows to a height of about 3 feet, and has yellow flowers with a purple base and heart-shaped leaves.

- Cottonseed oil is extracted from the small seeds of the cotton plant and used in shortenings, margarine, salad, and cooking oil.

- Because cotton is generally not considered a food crop, few precautions are taken by growers on the use and selection of pesticides and defoliants.

CAUTION: The oil should be considered unsafe for consumption or skin use. The seed, stem, and root of the cotton plant produce a substance called Gossypol, which suppresses sperm production in men. It has been used as an antifertility agent in China. The antifertility effect may become permanent. Twelve months after discontinuing the intake of Gossypol, more than 50% of the males still showed a sperm count of zero. Female animals are also affected by having aborted pregnancies. (Huang, Kee Chang. *The Pharmacology of Chinese Herbs*. CRC Press, 1993. p. 255)

EVENING PRIMROSE

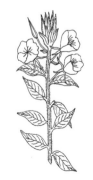

Botanical Name: *Oenothera biennis*
Family: *Onagraceae*

The oil is obtained from the seeds of the plant.

History and Information

- Evening primrose grows to a height of about 1–8 feet and has many fragrant yellow flowers that open at dusk to attract night-flying insects for pollination. The plant originated in North America and was exported to Europe during the 17th century.

- The American Indians made a preparation from the roots and applied it on their muscles to improve their strength. The roots were also used to treat obesity, hemorrhoids, and bruises.

- The seeds, flowers, leaves, and roots can be eaten cooked or raw, as in a salad. The roots taste similar to turnips.

- The oil contains a high amount of essential fatty acids.

Practical Uses

Helps premenstrual stress
Relieves menstrual pain, reduces inflammation
Skin care; moisturizing, soothing
The carrier/base oil is used to dilute essential oils in aromatherapy for massage oils and other formulations. For massage oils, it is best to mix 20% of evening primrose oil with another carrier oil.

Documented Properties

Analgesic, Antiarthritic, Anti-inflammatory, Antiscorbutic, Antispasmodic, Antitoxic, Astringent (*Mild*), Calmative, Depurative, Diuretic, Febrifuge, Hepatic, Hypotensor, Nervine, Stimulant, Tonic, Uplifting

FLAXSEED

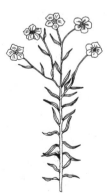

Botanical Name: *Linum usitatissimum*
Family: *Linaceae*

The oil is obtained from the seeds of the plant.

History and Information

- Flax has been cultivated before recorded history and, therefore, its place of origin is uncertain. The plant grows to a height of about 2 feet, and has sky-blue flowers and brown seeds.

- Cloths made of flax fiber were found in Egyptian burial chambers.

- In Switzerland, archaeologists discovered flaxseed and flax fiber cloth dated about 5000 B.C. For at least two centuries, the flax plant was one of the main sources of fabric for American clothing.

- Hippocrates mentioned the use of flaxseed to relieve inflammation of mucous membranes and abdominal pains.

- Emperor Charlemagne considered flaxseed so important to health that he issued a decree requiring its consumption.

- The oil was a folk remedy used for pleurisy, pneumonia, and cancer.

- Throughout history, flax has been used to maintain the health of animals. Farmers have reported that pregnant cows fed with flaxseed gave birth to healthier calves. When flaxseeds are added to the diets of pets, their fur coat improves.

- The oil is used in Europe for high-quality suntan and skin lotions, which nourish the skin with valuable essential fatty acids.

- In Germany, Dr. Johanna Budwig, a world-renowned holistic doctor, who studies and researches the effect of vegetable oils on the body, treats seriously ill patients by adding freshly pressed flaxseed oil to their diet.

- The unrefined fresh flax oil is a rich food source of both essential fatty acids. It contains 15 to 25% linoleic acid and 50 to 60% linolenic acid, which are necessary for good health. In addition, the oil is rich in lecithin and contains all of the essential amino acids and almost every known trace mineral. The oil spoils easily; therefore, to preserve the valuable properties, it is best to store it in the freezer.

- The seed has an oil content of 35%.

Practical Uses

Skin care
The carrier/base oil is used to dilute essential oils in aromatherapy for massage oils and other formulations.

Documented Properties

Anti-inflammatory, Antiseptic, Antitussive, Demulcent, Digestive, Emollient, Laxative, Purgative

GRAPESEED

Botanical Name: *Vitis vinifera*
Family: *Vitaceae*

The oil is obtained from the seeds of the fruit.

History and Information

- The grape plant is a climbing vine native to Asia. The vine grows to about 30 feet, and has green flowers that develop into sweet green or purple fruits.

- Grapeseed oil is produced from the residue of grapes that were pressed for wine. The oil is widely used in creams, massage oils, and on people who are allergic to other oils.

Practical Uses

General skin care
The carrier/base oil is used to dilute essential oils in aromatherapy for massage oils and other formulations. Grapeseed oil is a good massage oil that absorbs quickly into the skin.

HAZELNUT

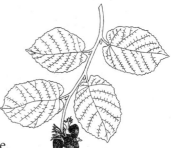

Botanical Name:
Corylus avellana
Family: *Betulaceae*

The oil is obtained from the nut of the tree.

History and Information

- Hazelnut is a deciduous tree native to Europe and Asia. The tree grows to a height of about 12–30 feet.

- The American Indians used the bark for hives, fevers, and wounds, and the twigs to expel intestinal parasites.

- Another name for hazelnut is filbert nut and cob nut. The nut is rich in oil, containing a 62% content.

Practical Uses

Skin care; moisturizes, softens, repairs dry and damaged skin

The carrier/base oil is used to dilute essential oils in aromatherapy for massage oils and other formulations.

Documented Properties

Antilithic, Aphrodisiac, Astringent (*Mild*), Parasiticide, Stomachic, Tonic

JOJOBA

Botanical Name: *Simmondsia chinensis*
Family: *Buxaceae*

The vegetable wax/oil is obtained from the beans of the shrub.

History and Information

- Jojoba is an evergreen shrub native to the southwestern United States and northern Mexico. The plant grows to a height of about 3–18 feet and has small leathery leaves. There are male and female plants. The male flowers are yellow; the female flowers are green and develop into olive-shaped fruits containing seeds inside. These seeds are called goat nut. Jojoba plants can live up to 200 years.

- The American Indians used jojoba oil for cooking and applied it to soothe their skin.

- Historically, jojoba oil has been used as a hair restorer.

- The oil is similar to sperm-whale oil and can be used as a substitute for it.

- The wax is used to make candles, furniture polish and floor wax, and in industry to lubricate machinery since it can withstand high temperatures. The oil is added as an ingredient in shampoos, moisturizers, sunscreens, and hair conditioners. Jojoba oil is stable and, if stored properly, can last for many years without spoiling.

Practical Uses

Skin care; moisturizes and softens dry skin; helps with stretch marks
Suntanning oil for those who burn easily in the sun
Scalp and hair care
The carrier/base oil is used to dilute essential oils in aromatherapy for massage oils and other formulations. For massage oils, it is best to mix 50% of jojoba oil with another carrier oil before adding the essential oils.

Documented Properties

Anti-inflammatory, Antiseptic, Emollient

KIWIFRUIT SEED

Botanical Name: *Actinidia chinensis*
Family: *Actinidiaceae*

The oil is obtained from the fruit and seeds of the vine.

History and Information

- The kiwi is a climbing vine native to China, and has heart-shaped leaves and white flowers. The plant is also known as Chinese gooseberry.

- The largest producers of kiwifruit are New Zealand and France.

- The oil is unsuitable as a cooking oil because it becomes unstable when heated.

Practical Uses

Skin care

The carrier/base oil is used to dilute essential oils in aromatherapy for massage oils and other formulations.

Documented Properties

Regenerator (*Skin*), Tonic

KUKUI NUT

Botanical Name: *Aleurites moluccana*
Family: *Euphorbiaceae*

The oil is obtained from the nut of the tree.

History and Information

- Kukui nut is an evergreen tree native to Asia. The tree grows to a height of about 70 feet and has white flowers that develop into nuts. The kukui nut tree is also referred to as varnish tree, candlenut tree, and candleberry tree. Kukui is the official tree of the State of Hawaii.

- The Polynesian people use the nuts as a food source and fuel for their torches; they also use the oil as a laxative and the wood of the tree for making canoes.

- In Indonesia, the oil is used to treat hair loss and soften calluses.

- In China, the oil is massaged into the scalp to stimulate hair growth.

- Kukui nuts are also known as candlenuts, since they are used as candles.

- The nuts are roasted and eaten. For some people, they act as a strong purgative. Kukui oil is also known as lumbag oil.

Practical Uses

Skin care; balances, rejuvenates and softens the skin
The carrier/base oil is used to dilute essential oils in aromatherapy for massage oils and other formulations.

MACADAMIA NUT

Botanical Name: *Macadamia integrifolia*
Family: *Protoceae*

The oil is obtained from the nut of the tree.

History and Information

- Macadamia is an evergreen tree native to Australia. The tree grows to a height of about 30–70 feet. Macadamia was first domesticated in Australia in the mid-1800's.

- The nut, also known as queensland nut and Australian nut, has an oil content of 71%.

Practical Uses

Skin care; softens and restores the skin
The carrier/base oil is used to dilute essential oils in aromatherapy for massage oils and other formulations.

MANGO

Botanical Name: *Mangifera indica*
Family: *Anacardiaceae*

The oil is obtained from the kernel of the fruit.

History and Information

- Mango is a fast-growing evergreen tree native to Asia. It reaches a height of about 100 feet, and has small fragrant clusters of pink or light green flowers that develop into edible fruits. The mango has 210 varieties and is often referred to as the "queen of tropical fruits."

- The tree has been cultivated since 2000 B.C. in India.

- All parts of the tree are used; the leaves provide a sour flavoring for foods, and the fruit is eaten fresh, dried, or pickled.

- The trunk, branches, and unripe fruit contain a sap that is a skin irritant.

Practical Uses

Skin care; hair care
The carrier/base oil is used to dilute essential oils in aromatherapy for massage oils and other formulations. For massage oils, it is best to mix 20% of mango oil with another carrier oil before adding the essential oils.

Documented Properties

Anthelmintic, Astringent

MANGOSTEEN (Kokum Butter)

Botanical Name: *Garcinia mangostana*
Family: *Guttiferae*

The butter is obtained from the kernel of the fruit of the tree.

History and Information

- Mangosteen is a slow-growing tree native to Asia. The tree grows to a height of about 30 feet, and has large, leathery, thick glossy leaves, large pink flowers, and an edible fruit. The fruit is about the size of an orange and has a thick hard rind with white flesh inside. The tree can yield more than one thousand fruits in a season.

- In China, the dried fruits are used for dysentery and made into a ointment for skin problems.

Practical Uses

Soothing and moisturizing to the skin

Documented Properties

Skin moisturizer; skin problems

NEEM

Botanical Name: *Azadirachta indica*
Family: *Meliaceae*

The oil is obtained from the seeds of the tree.

History and Information

- Neem is native to Asia. The tree is evergreen except in freezing temperature regions. It grows to a height of about 100 feet, and has white or yellow fragrant flowers and a yellow fruit with a seed inside. Neem is also known as nim or margosa.

- The neem tree is considered sacred in India.

- The first reported use of neem was by the ancient Indian Harappa culture around 2500

B.C. For centuries, the oil has been used in Asia for skin and hair care, the bark extract for mouth and gum inflammations, and the leaves as an insecticide.

- In countries where the neem grows, every part of the tree is used. A resin is produced when the trunk is wounded. The leaves are added to animal feed for their high protein content; the seeds and leaves yield an insect repellent; the fruits are sweet-tasting and have an olive-like appearance.

- The tree contains the chemical component, azadirachtin, which interferes with the metamorphosis of insect larvae. Many leaf-chewing insects find the tree leaves so repulsive that they would rather die of starvation than eat the leaves. (*Neem, a Tree for Solving Global Problems.* National Academy Press, 1992)

- Farmers and food merchants add neem to grains in storage to prevent insect infestation.

- The seeds yield approximately 40% oil. The oil is an ingredient in toothpastes, lotions, and soaps. The unrefined oil contains sulfur compounds, which contribute to the pungent odor that is similar to garlic.

Practical Uses

Skin care

Documented Properties

Antibacterial, Antifungal, Anti-inflammatory, Insecticide, Tonic

OLIVE

Botanical Name: *Olea europaea*
Family: *Oleaceae*

The oil is obtained from the fruit of the tree.

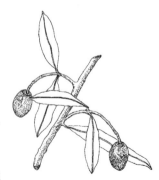

History and Information

- Olive is an evergreen tree native to the Mediterranean region. The tree reaches a height of about 25–40 feet and has fragrant clusters of white flowers. Olive trees are slow to mature, requiring 10 years to start to bear fruit, and 30 years for a sizable crop to be produced. The trees may reach an age of 1500 years.

- The first historical mention of the olive occurred in Egypt in the 17th century B.C.

- The olive was an ancient symbol of peace and prosperity.

- Throughout history, olive oil was the most important of all the vegetable oils. Italy, Spain, Greece, and France produce the finest quality of olive oil.

- As a folk remedy, the leaves were used to lower blood pressure and blood sugar levels.

- The first pressing of the finest selected olives is called extra virgin oil, which is considered the top grade. Virgin oil is considered the second-best grade and pure olive oil is the third. The pure olive oil is extracted from the pulp and pits left over from the other pressings; it is generally produced by the use of heat and high pressure, solvents, bleaching, and deodorizing.

- Olive oil oxidizes less rapidly than other oils; therefore, it has a longer shelf-life. The olive has an oil content of 20%.

Practical Uses

Skin care
Due to its thickness, olive oil does not absorb readily into the skin and is best not to be used as a carrier oil.

Documented Properties

Antipruritic, Cholagogue, Demulcent, Emollient, Laxative, Relaxant, Vulnerary

PALM & PALM KERNEL

Botanical Name: *Elaeis guineensis*
Family: *Arecaceae*

Palm oil is obtained from the fruit of the tree. Palm kernel oil is obtained from the seeds.

History and Information

- Palm is native to Africa. The tree grows to a height of about 70 feet and has clusters of two hundred to three hundred flowers. The fruits are plum-like in appearance.

- Palm oil has been used for more than 5000 years.

- The tree yields more oil per acre than any other vegetable oil plant. Two types of oil are produced from the palm tree; both are quite similar to coconut oil and are used in soaps, candles, ointments, margarine, shortenings, and cooking. Palm oil is the second most produced oil in the world—the first being soybean oil. The unrefined oil is reddish brown and can rapidly turn rancid.

- During the 1700's, palm oil was used in Britain as a hand cream.

- Palm oil is solid at room temperature.

- Both the fruit and seed have an oil content of 35%, and are especially rich in carotene.

- The tree yields a sap that is used, in Africa, as a laxative. The fermented sap is made into a wine taken by nursing mothers to increase lactation.

Practical Uses

Skin care

Documented Properties

Analgesic, Antidote, Aphrodisiac, Diuretic, Galactagogue, Laxative, Vulnerary

PASSION FRUIT SEED

Botanical Name: *Passiflora incarnata*
Family: *Passifloraceae*

The oil is obtained from the kernels and fruit of the vine.

History and Information

- Passion fruit is a climbing vine native to America. The plant reaches a height of about 30 feet, and has flowers approximately 2 inches wide with white or lavender petals. Passionflower bears an edible egg-shaped fruit that is about 3 inches long.

- Throughout the years, the herb was most commonly used for nervous conditions.

- The American Indians used the leaves and the root as a poultice for injuries and boils, and as a tea for calming their nerves.

- The leaves of the plant are an ingredient in many European medicines for nervous disorders.

Practical Uses

Skin care; soothing
The carrier/base oil is used to dilute essential oils in aromatherapy for massage oils and other formulations.

PEANUT

Botanical Name: *Arachis hypogaea*
Family: *Fabaceae*

The oil is obtained from the "nuts" of the plant.

History and Information

- Peanut is native to Central and South America. The plant grows to a height of about a foot and has yellow flowers. After becoming pollinated, the stalk bearing the flowers pushes the pods into the soil. The pods remain there until maturity. The peanut plant is a member of the bean family rather than the nut. The plant grows in warm climates around the world. Peanut is also known as groundnut.

- In China, peanuts are used to stop bleeding and increase lactation in nursing mothers.

Practical Uses

Skin care

Documented Properties

Galactagogue, Hemostatic

PECAN

Botanical Name: *Carya illinoinensis*
Family: *Juglandaceae*

The oil is obtained from the nut of the tree.

History and Information

- Pecan is native to North America and belongs to the walnut family. The tree grows to a height of about 100–170 feet and produces a thin-shelled nut. Pecan is the official tree in Texas.

- The nuts were a food staple of the American Indians.

- Pecans have a high oil content of 71%.

Practical Uses

Skin care
The carrier/base oil is used to dilute essential oils in aromatherapy for massage oils and other formulations.

PINE NUT

Botanical Name: *Pinus edulis, P. pinea*
Family: *Pinaceae*

The oil is obtained from the nut of the tree.

History and Information

- The *Pinus pinea* species is native to the Mediterranean region and referred to as the Italian stone pine. The tree grows to a height of about 80 feet, and has needle-like leaves and nuts inside the cones. Generally, the tree does not bear any edible nuts until its fifteenth year when cultivated and about the twenty-fifth year when growing in the wild. The nuts take approximately 3 years to ripen. The species of *Pinus edulis* is native to America and grows to a height of about 50 feet.

- Pine nuts are found in the cones of certain pine trees. They are also referred to as pignolia, pine seed, and piñon. More than one hundred seeds may be in a single cone.

- The nuts have been prized as a delicacy over the years especially in China and Japan. Many Mediterranean dishes contain pine nuts.

- The nut has an oil content of 55% and contains the highest amount of protein of all the nuts.

Practical Uses

Skin care; soothing and healing to the skin tissues
The carrier/base oil is used to dilute essential oils in aromatherapy for massage oils and other formulations. The oil is light in texture and absorbs readily into the skin.

Documented Properties

Tonic

PISTACHIO NUT

Botanical Name: *Pistacia vera*
Family: *Anacardiaceae*

The oil is obtained from the nut of the tree.

History and Information

- Pistachio nut is native to Asia. The tree grows to a height of about 30–40 feet and can live to approximately 1500 years. The male and female flowers are produced on different trees. Pistachio is related to the poison ivy, poison oak, poison sumac, mango, and the cashew nut tree.

- The nut contains an oil content of 54% and is rich in iron. The oil is used in food flavorings and cosmetics.

Practical Uses

Skin care; moisturizing
The carrier/base oil is used to dilute essential oils in aromatherapy for massage oils and other formulations.

Documented Properties

Analgesic, Anticoagulant, Antitoxic, Aphrodisiac, Digestive, Hepatic, Tonic

PUMPKINSEED

Botanical Name: *Cucurbita pepo*
Family: *Cucurbitaceae*

The oil is obtained from the seeds of the plant.

History and Information

- The pumpkin is native to the Americas. The climbing plant reaches a length of about 30 feet, and has large leaves, fragrant yellow-orange flowers, and orange fruits. Pumpkins are the largest fruits in the plant kingdom.

- In Oriental medicine, a tea made from the seeds, taken over a period of time, is said to help reduce swellings of the legs, ankles, and abdomen.

- In Latin America, Africa, and India, the seeds are used to expel intestinal worms. Some European physicians recommend pumpkin seeds to prevent prostate problems in men. The seeds contain nutrients known to be components of the male hormone.

- In China, the roasted seeds are eaten to promote longevity.

- The seed has an oil content of 46%. Most of the oil is produced in Austria and popularly used to flavor food.

Practical Uses

Skin care
The carrier/base oil is used to dilute essential oils in aromatherapy for massage oils and other formulations. Due to the pumpkinseed oil's sticky nature, it is best to mix 20% of the oil with another carrier oil.

Documented Properties

Anti-inflammatory, Stomachic, Tonic, Vermifuge, Vulnerary

RICE BRAN

Botanical Name: *Oryza sativa*
Family: *Poaceae*

The oil is obtained from the grain of the plant.

History and Information

- Rice is native to Asia. The plant grows to a height of about 2–4 feet, and has narrow blade-like leaves and grains encased in husks.

- Rice has been a food staple since 2500 BC.
- Rice bran is said to contain a substance that helps to prevent deposits in the arteries.
- The bran has an oil content of only 10%.

Practical Uses

Skin care; soothing
The carrier/base oil is used to dilute essential oils in aromatherapy for massage oils and other formulations. The oil has a light texture and readily absorbs into the skin.

Documented Properties

Antidiarrhoeic, Depurative, Hypotensive, Tonic

ROSE HIP SEED

Botanical Name: *Rosa rubiginosa*
Family: *Rosaceae*

The oil is obtained from the hips and seeds of the bush.

History and Information

- Rose is native to the Mediterranean region. There are many varieties of the rose bush that grow to various heights and produce fragrant flowers ranging in colors.
- Since the beginning of time, the rose has been considered the most valuable flower for beautifying and restoring health to the skin.

Practical Uses

Skin care, moisturizing, skin regenerator, reduces wrinkles
The carrier/base oil is used to dilute essential oils in aromatherapy for massage oils and other formulations.

SAFFLOWER

Botanical Name: *Carthamus tinctorius*
Family: *Asteraceae*

The oil is obtained from the seeds of the plant.

History and Information

- Safflower is native to India. The plant grows about 3 feet high and has orange-yellow flowers.
- The historical use of safflower oil dates back to the ancient times when it was used by the Egyptian pharaohs for cooking.
- During the Middle Ages, juiced safflower seeds mixed with sweetened water was a recommended drink when suffering from respiratory ailments and constipation.
- Safflower oil was introduced experimentally in the United States as an oil crop in 1925.
- The flowers yield a red and yellow dye, the seeds produce an oil, and the leaves are eaten as a vegetable. The red dye has been used since ancient times to color cloths, especially silk, and in makeup, such as rouge. The yellow dye is used as a food coloring agent. The seed has an oil content of 59%. Approximately 75% of the oil consists of linoleic acid, which is an essential fatty acid that plays an important nutritional role in the body. Because it is rich in unsaturated fatty acids, safflower is one of the most popular oils used as a salad and cooking oil. It has also been noted for its ability to slow down digestion and allow the food to combine with the digestive enzymes for proper assimilation.

Practical Uses

Skin care
The carrier/base oil is used to dilute essential oils in aromatherapy for massage oils and other formulations.

Documented Properties

Analgesic, Depurative, Diaphoretic, Digestive, Diuretic, Febrifuge, Hypotensor, Regenerator, Stimulant (*Uterine*), Tonic

SEA BUCKTHORN

Botanical Name: *Hippophae rhamnoides*
Family: *Elaeagnaceae*

The oil is obtained from the berries of the shrub.

History and Information

- Sea buckthorn is native to Europe and Asia. The shrub grows to a height of about 30 feet and has clusters of yellow flowers that develop into small orange berries.

- The people of Nepal eat the berries raw or preserved.

- The red dye from the fruit is used by women in Asia to color their face and lips. A yellow dye is made from the plant and roots.

Practical Uses

Warming; improves circulation
Relaxing
Mood uplifting
Loosens tight muscles
Softens and heals the skin

SESAME

Botanical Name: *Sesamum indicum*
Family: *Pedaliaceae*

The oil is obtained from the seeds of the plant.

History and Information

- Sesame is native to Africa and Asia. The plant grows to a height of about 3–6 feet, and has white or pink tubular flowers with purple spots. The color of the seeds can be white, yellow, red, brown, or black. There are thirty-seven species of the plant. Sesame is also referred to as sim-sim. Sesame oil is also known as benne oil, gingle oil, and teel oil.

- The seeds and leaves have been eaten in Africa and India since ancient times. It is probably the oldest crop grown for its oil. Records of the production of sesame seeds date back to 1600 B.C.

- The name sesame was included on a list of Egyptian medicinal preparations recorded on papyrus dated about 1550 B.C.

- Women in ancient Babylonia used sesame seeds and honey to increase their vitality for lovemaking and fertility.

- Sesame has been the primary cooking oil in Africa and Asia.

- In Oriental medicine, a tea, made from the seeds, is consumed two to three times daily to promote an abundant supply of milk in nursing mothers, improve eyesight, and darken the hair. In China, the seeds are cooked in water and made into a soup to relieve toothaches and swollen gums. A paste, made from the seeds, is recommended for hemorrhoids and to heal sores. The flower and leaf infusions are said to improve hair growth.

- The seed has an oil content of 49%. It is more stable and oxidizes less than other oils when heated. The oil has a shelf-life of several years. The raw seeds produce a light-colored oil and the roasted seeds yield a darker colored oil.

Practical Uses

Skin care; moisturizing, soothing
Hair and scalp care
The carrier/base oil is used to dilute essential oils in aromatherapy for massage oils and other formulations.

Documented Properties

Emollient, Galactagogue, Laxative, Sun Protectant, Tonic

SHEA BUTTER

Botanical Name: *Butyrosperum parkii*
Family: *Sapotaceae*

The butter is obtained from the nut kernels of the tree.

History and Information

- Shea is native to Africa. The tree grows to a height of about 70 feet and has white flowers with a sweet fragrance. The fruit is brown with a large white kernel inside.

- In Africa, the butter is used for food and in body care products. It is also employed as a massage oil for sore muscles, burns, and bruises.

- In Japan, shea butter is used as a substitute for dairy butter.

- The seeds contain 50% fat content. The bark yields a reddish gum called gutta shea. Shea oil is made from the raw kernels while shea butter is produced from the roasted kernels that are put through a process. The butter is also known as African butter and karite butter.

Practical Uses

Skin and hair moisturizer
Suntan creme
Massage creme

SISYMBRIUM

Botanical Name: *Sisymbrium officinale*
Family: *Brassicaceae*

The oil is obtained from the seeds of the plant.

History and Information

- Sisymbrium is native to North America and Europe. The plant is also known as hedge mustard, which is a common weed that grows up to 4 feet high and has small yellow flowers. The seeds develop from the flowers and resemble mustard seeds.

- Sisymbrium is known for its beautifying properties. Roman women had their servants massage rose and sisymbrium oil on their bodies after bathing.

- In some areas of India, sisymbrium seed infusions are used to treat many skin diseases. In other countries, the seeds are used in facial masks to improve the skin's complexion.

- In Britain, the plant is eaten as a vegetable.

Practical Uses

Skin care; softens the skin, improves the complexion; reduces wrinkles
The carrier/base oil is used to dilute essential oils in aromatherapy for massage oils and other formulations. For massage oils, it is best to mix 20% of sisymbrium oil with another carrier oil before adding the essential oils. Sisymbrium oil absorbs into the skin very quickly, leaving no oily residue.

Documented Properties

Diuretic, Expectorant, Stomachic

SOYBEAN

Botanical Name: *Soja hispida*
Family: *Fabaceae*

The oil is obtained from the bean of the plant.

History and Information

- Soybean is a bushy plant native to Asia. The plant grows to a height of about 6 feet, and has small white or purple flowers.

- The soybean plant was first cultivated in China around the 11th century B.C. Today, it is one of the world's most important sources of protein.

- The beans are rich in estrogen, and could inhibit fertility or help replace estrogen in postmenopausal women.

- Soybean oil contains 2% lecithin and beneficial essential fatty acids. Choline, found in lecithin, is needed for the proper function of the brain and liver. In addition, choline enables the body to utilize cholesterol and fats, and prevents deposits of cholesterol in the arterial linings.

- Since the beans only contain 17% oil, high temperatures and toxic solvents are commonly used to extract the oil. Soybean oil is used in cooking, margarine, shortening, salad dressing, and for industrial products.

Practical Uses

The carrier/base oil is used to dilute essential oils in aromatherapy for massage oils and other formulations. For massage oils, it is best to mix 10% of soybean oil with another carrier oil before adding the essential oils.

Documented Properties

Detoxifier, Diuretic, Estrogenic, Febrifuge, Stimulant, Tonic

SUNFLOWER

Botanical Name: *Helianthus annuus*
Family: *Asteraceae*

The oil is obtained from the seeds of the plant.

History and Information

- Sunflower is native to America. The plant grows to a height of about 6–15 feet, and has a tall hairy stem and large orange-yellow flowers that look similar to a large daisy. There are 110 varieties of sunflower plants and they belong to the daisy family.

- Sunflowers were first grown as an oil crop in Bavaria in 1725, then in France in 1787.

- Gypsies used the fresh leaves and flowers of the plant to treat malaria.

- The Inca Indians of Peru worshipped the sunflower. The American Indians highly regarded the plant; they used the oil as a tonic for the hair and brewed the flowers to relieve congestion and as a remedy for malaria.

- A tea brewed from the flowers was used in Europe as a remedy for chest congestion and coughs.

- The czars of Russia fed their soldiers 2 pounds of sunflower seeds as part of their daily food rations.

- Chickens lay more eggs when sunflower seeds are added to their diet.

- The seed has an oil content of 47% and contains high amounts of essential fatty acids. The oil is used to make candles and soaps, the burnt stems for potash, and the leaves for an herbal tobacco.

Practical Uses

Skin care
The carrier/base oil is used to dilute essential oils in aromatherapy for massage oils and other formulations.

Documented Properties

Antisclerotic, Antiseptic, Aphrodisiac, Diuretic, Emollient, Expectorant, Insecticidal, Sudorific

WALNUT

Botanical Name: *Juglans regia*
Family: *Juglandaceae*

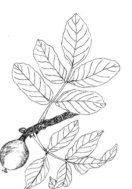

The oil is obtained from the nuts of the tree.

History and Information

- Walnut is a deciduous tree native to America, Europe, and Asia. It grows to a height of about 100 feet. The dark green leaves are glossy and oval-shaped; the female flowers are green and the male flowers are yellowish-green in catkins. The nuts are hard shelled.

- In an ancient Chinese herbal, walnut was described as promoting circulation, darkening the hair, and making the skin smooth. It was used to relieve stomach acid and excessive urination.

- In Ayurvedic medicine, walnuts are considered to be a brain tonic.

- The American Indians juiced the hulls as a remedy to rid their animals of parasites. The crushed green hulls were also used to stupefy fish so that they could be easily caught.

- Until the end of the 18th century, European households drank walnut milk as a substitute for dairy milk. The nuts were finely powdered and soaked in water to create this nourishing drink.

- Gypsies have traditionally used the nut hulls and tree roots to make dyes; theatrical performers have also used them to stain their skin dark brown.

- Many Europeans substitute olive oil with walnut oil. In southern Europe, walnut oil has long been popular for cooking. France is said to make the finest-quality oil, which accounts for approximately 33% of the country's total oil production.

- In Germany, a tea made from walnut leaves is given daily to children for 2–6 months to alleviate skin problems.

- In China, the nuts are used as a laxative and pain reliever.

- When the bark is tapped in the spring, it yields a sweet sap similar to maple syrup.

- The green rind of the walnut has been used in many applications, such as a fungicide for agriculture, in a poultice for ringworm, and as a source of iodine for individuals deficient in it. The inner bark and leaves have been used for skin problems, gout, colic, impotence, and to expel worms.

- The nut has a rich oil content of 60%. The oil is used in tanning lotions. The wood is used in making valuable furniture.

Practical Uses

Skin care
The carrier/base oil is used to dilute essential oils in aromatherapy for massage oils and other formulations.

Documented Properties

Analgesic, Antigalactagogue, Anti-inflammatory, Antilithic, Antispasmodic, Aperitive, Astringent, Digestive, Moisturizing (*Lungs*), Parasiticide, Tonic, Vasoconstrictor, Vermifuge, Vulnerary

WHEAT GERM

Botanical Name: *Triticum vulgare*
Family: *Poaceae*

The oil is obtained from the grain of the plant.

History and Information

- Wheat has been one of the most important food staples worldwide. The plant belongs to the grass family and grows to a height of about 2–4 feet.

- Wheat germ oil contains valuable essential fatty acids; the linoleic acid content is approximately 58%. It is also a rich source of vitamins, especially vitamin E, a natural antioxidant that helps prolong the shelf-life of any blend to which it is added.

- The wheat germ has an oil content of only 10%.

Practical Uses

Skin care
The carrier/base oil is used to dilute essential oils in aromatherapy for massage oils and other formulations. For massage oils, it is best to mix 10% of wheat germ oil with another carrier oil before adding the essential oils.

Documented Properties

Galactagogue, Tonic

CHAPTER 3

Essential Oils

Essential oils are the precious essences extracted from herbs, flowers, and trees. These wonderful, pure, and fragrant oils contain a natural living substance known as the "essence," which is the concentrated power and vital life force of the plant.

The following essential oils are covered in this chapter:

Ajowan
Allspice (*Pimento*)
Ambrette Seed
Amyris
Angelica Root
Angelica Seed
Anise
Anise (*Star*)
Basil (*Sweet*)
Bay (*Sweet*)
Bay (*West Indian*)
Benzoin
Bergamot
Birch (*Sweet*)
Birch (*White*)
Bois de Rose
Cabreuva
Cade
Cajeput
Calamint (*Catnip*)
Calamus (*Sweet Flag*)
Camphor
Camphor (*Borneol*)
Cananga
Caraway
Cardamom
Carnation (*Clove Pink*)
Cascarilla Bark
Cassia
Cassie
Cedarwood
Cedarwood (*Atlas*)
Celery

Chamomile (*German*)
Chamomile (*Moroccan*)
Chamomile (*Roman*)
Champaca Flower
Champaca Leaf
Cinnamon Bark
Cinnamon Leaf
Citronella
Clary Sage
Clove Bud
Clove Leaf
Clove Stem
Coffee
Copaiba
Coriander
Cornmint
Costus
Cubeb
Cumin
Cyperus (*Cypriol*)
Cypress
Dill Seed
Dill Weed
Elecampane
Elemi
Eucalyptus
Eucalyptus Citriodora
Eucalyptus Radiata
Fennel
Fir, Douglas
Fir, Grand
Fir Needles
Fir, Silver

Fir Balsam Needles
Fir Balsam Resin
Frankincense
   (*Olibanum*)
Galangal
Galbanum
Gardenia
Geranium
Ginger
Gingergrass
Goldenrod
Grapefruit
Guaiacwood
Helichrysum (*Everlasting, Immortelle*)
Hops
Hyssop
Hyssop Decumbens
Jasmine
Juniper Berries
Labdanum (*Cistus, Rock Rose*)
Lantana
Larch
Lavandin
Lavender
Ledum Groenlandicum
Lemon
Lemon Verbena
Lemongrass
Leptospermum (*New Zealand Tea Tree*)
Lime

Linden Blossom
Litsea Cubeba
Lovage
Mandarin
Marjoram (*Spanish*)
Marjoram (*Sweet*)
Massoia Bark
Mastic
Melissa (*Lemon Balm*)
Mimosa
Monarda
Mugwort (*Armoise*)
Myrrh
Myrtle
Neroli
Niaouli
Nutmeg
Orange
Oregano
Orris Root
Osmanthus
Palmarosa
Parsley
Patchouli
Pennyroyal
Pepper (*Black*)
Peppermint
Peru Balsam
Petitgrain
Pine
Ravensara Anisata
   (*Havozo Bark*)
Ravensara Aromatica

Rhododendron	Savory	Tangerine	Turmeric
Rose	Spearmint	Tarragon (*Estragon*)	Valerian
Rosemary	Spikenard	Tea Tree	Vanilla
Rue	Spruce	Temple Orange	Vetiver
Saffron	Spruce-Hemlock	Terebinth	Violet
Sage	Spruce-Sitka	Thuja (*Cedar Leaf*)	Wintergreen
Sage (*Spanish*)	St. John's Wort	Thyme	Wormwood
Sandalwood	Styrax (*Liquidamber* or	Tobacco Leaf	Yarrow
Santolina (*Lavender Cotton*)	*Storax*)	Tolu Balsam	Ylang-Ylang
Sassafras	Tagetes	Tonka Bean	Zanthoxylum
	Tangelo	Tuberose	

AJOWAN

Botanical Name: *Trachyspermum ammi, T. copticum*
Family: *Apiaceae*

The essential oil is obtained from the seeds of the plant.

History and Information

- Ajowan is native to Asia. The plant grows to a height of about 2 feet.

- The herb is utilized in Ayurvedic medicine in India to treat cholera and other intestinal problems.

- The seeds are used in curry powder as a seasoning for food.

Practical Uses

Heating; improves circulation
Promotes a restful sleep
Soothes sore and tight muscles

Documented Properties

Antibacterial, Antifungal, Antiseptic (*Strong*), Antiviral, Aphrodisiac, Carminative, Parasiticide, Tonic

CAUTION: Ajowan oil is moderately toxic; use small amounts. Ajowan can irritate the skin and should be either avoided or used with extra care by people with sensitive skin.

ALLSPICE (*Pimento*)

Botanical Name: *Pimenta dioica, P. officinalis*
Family: *Myrtaceae*

The essential oil is obtained from the twigs, leaves, and dried unripe berries of the tree.

History and Information

- Allspice is an evergreen tree native to the West Indies and Central America. The tree grows to a height of about 30–70 feet, and has leathery leaves and small white flowers that develop into aromatic berries, which turn black when ripe.

- In Guatemala, the crushed allspice berries are applied to painful muscles and joints.

- Allspice leaf oil is similar in composition to clove leaf oil, both containing high amounts of eugenol.

Practical Uses

Warming; improves circulation
Improves digestion
Purifying; helps in the reduction of cellulite
Calms the nerves, removes stress; promotes a restful sleep
Vapors open the sinus and breathing passages
Mood uplifting
Loosens tight muscles, lessens pain

Documented Properties

Analgesic, Antidepressant, Antioxidant, Antiseptic, Aphrodisiac, Carminative, Digestive, Rubefacient, Stomachic, Tonic, Tranquilizer

Aromatherapy Methods of Use: Application, aroma lamp, diffusor, inhaler, light bulb ring, massage, mist spray, steam inhalation

CAUTION: Allspice oil can irritate the skin and should be either avoided or used with extra care by people with sensitive skin. Pimento berry oil is milder to the skin than the leaf oil.

AMBRETTE SEED

Botanical Name: *Abelmoschus moschatus, Hibiscus abelmoschus*
Family: *Malvaceae*

The essential oil is obtained from the seeds of the shrub.

History and Information

● Ambrette is a evergreen shrub native to Asia. The bushy plant grows to a height of about 5 feet, and has large yellow and purple flowers. The fruit is an oblong seedpod that splits at the tip when it matures. The seeds smell like musk.

● In China, ambrette seeds have been used as a remedy for headaches, the root for fever and coughs, and the flowers for the skin.

● In Central America, the seeds are chewed to ease the stomach, calm the nerves, and for diuretic purposes. The seeds are placed topically on snakebites and a seed infusion is taken internally.

● In the Middle East, the seeds are used to flavor foods and coffee.

● The oil is an ingredient in cosmetics, perfumery, food flavorings, soft drinks, and alcoholic beverages.

Practical Uses

Calming; relieves nervous tension and reduces stress
Mood uplifting
Lessens aches and pains
Healing and moisturizing to the skin

Documented Properties

Analgesic, Antispasmodic, Aphrodisiac, Carminative, Diuretic, Nervine, Sedative, Stimulant, Stomachic

Aromatherapy Methods of Use: Application, aroma lamp, bath, inhaler, light bulb ring, massage, mist spray

CAUTION: Ambrette seed is phototoxic. Avoid exposure to direct sunlight several hours after applying the oil on the skin.

AMYRIS

Botanical Name: *Amyris balsamifera, Schimmelia oleifera*
Family: *Rutaceae*

The essential oil is obtained from the wood chips of the tree.

History and Information

● Amyris is an evergreen tree native to the West Indies and Central America. The tree grows to about 60 feet high and has clusters of white flowers that develop into an edible black-bluish fruit.

● Amyris is also known as West Indian sandalwood. It is commonly used to adulterate the true sandalwood oil and as a fixative in perfumery.

● The wood burns like a candle and is called candlewood.

Practical Uses

Cooling
Calming; reduces stress and tension; releases anxiety; promotes a peaceful state
Helps to deepen the breathing
Reviving; improves mental clarity
Loosens tight muscles
Used as a fixative to hold the scent of a fragrance

Documented Properties

Antiphlogistic, Antiseptic, Antispasmodic, Aphrodisiac, Balsamic, Expectorant, Fixative, Hypotensive, Lymphatic Decongestant, Sedative, Tonic (*Heart*)

Aromatherapy Methods of Use: Application, aroma lamp, bath, fragrancing, inhaler, light bulb ring, massage, mist spray, steam inhalation, steam and sauna room

ANGELICA ROOT & ANGELICA SEED

Botanical Name: *Angelica archangelica, A. officinalis*
Family: *Apiaceae*

Angelica root essential oil is obtained from the roots of the plant. Angelica seed essential oil is obtained from the seeds.

History and Information

- Angelica is native to Europe. The plant grows to about 6 feet in height and has clusters of yellow-green flowers.

- Paracelsus, the Swiss physician, used angelica during an epidemic in the 16th century.

- During the plague of 1665, the stems were chewed to prevent infection. The seeds and roots were burned to disinfect the air. The roots were also dried, powdered, and mixed with vinegar to disinfect linen and clothing when washing.

- The American Indians used angelica as an expectorant for respiratory congestion and tuberculosis, a tonic to recover from illness, and to expel worms.

- In Chinese medicine, angelica is used to correct menstrual irregularities, promote female fertility, and as a tonic for the liver.

- In Europe, the plant has been used as a remedy for coughs, colds, stomach problems, and as a blood purifier.

- In Asia, angelica is a highly regarded herb that is mainly used as a remedy for females who have menopause or menstrual problems.

- Both the seeds and roots yield an essential oil. The seeds produce a greater oil content and the root oil has a stronger odor. Angelica oil is highly valued as a fragrance in perfumes, and is used as a flavoring ingredient in foods, soft drinks, and liqueurs. All parts of the plant are edible: the shoots are added to a salad, the stalks are eaten like celery or candied as a confectionery, the roots are steamed as vegetables, and the seeds are used to flavor baked goods.

Practical Uses

Cooling
Improves digestion; soothes the intestines, relieves nausea
Calming; reduces stress
Vapors open the sinus and breathing passages; deepens breathing
Improves mental clarity and alertness; helps one to dream; helpful for meditation
Relieves aches, pains, and menstrual discomfort

Documented Properties

Analgesic, Antibacterial, Antifungal, Anti-inflammatory, Antirheumatic, Antiseptic, Antispasmodic, Antiviral, Aperitive, Aphrodisiac, Carminative, Cephalic, Depurative, Diaphoretic, Digestive, Diuretic, Emmenagogue, Estrogenic, Expectorant, Febrifuge, Hepatic, Healing (*Skin*), Nervine, Revitalizing, Stimulant (*Uterine; Nerves*), Stomachic, Sudorific, Tonic

Aromatherapy Methods of Use: Application, aroma lamp, bath, diffusor, inhaler, light bulb ring, massage, mist spray, steam inhalation, steam and sauna room

CAUTION: Due to the toxicity of the oil, use small amounts. Angelica root is phototoxic. Avoid exposure to direct sunlight several hours after applying the oil on the skin.

ANISE

Botanical Name: *Anisum officinalis, Pimpinella anisum*
Family: *Apiaceae*

The essential oil is obtained from the plant.

History and Information

- Anise is native to the Mediterranean area. The plant reaches a height of about 2 feet and has small white flowers.

- During biblical times, anise was highly valued and used by the Romans to pay their taxes. When the Romans discovered that the seeds of anise helped the digestion, they used them in special cakes served after their large banquets.

- The Egyptians grew large amounts of anise for cooking, teas, and medicines.

- Hippocrates used the herb to clear mucous from the respiratory system.

- Theophrastus, the father of botany, wrote that anise, kept near the bed at night, promoted sweet dreams.

- Pliny, the Roman herbalist, recommended chewing anise as a breath freshener and digestive aid. Today, the seeds are chewed in India for those same reasons.

- In 1305, King Edward I declared anise a taxable commodity. The resulting taxes supplied funds to repair the London bridge.

- The Aztec Indians chewed the seeds to relieve flatulence.

- In the 16th century, Europeans discovered that mice were attracted to anise and used it as bait in mousetraps.

- The American Indians made a tea from the leaves and flowers for a cough remedy.

- The seeds yield 2–3% essential oil, which is widely used in beverages, baking, foods, confectionery candy (licorice), cough drops, and liqueurs. Powdered anise seed is used to flavor horse and cattle feed.

Practical Uses

Improves digestion; soothes the intestines, relieves flatulence and aerophagy
Calming, relaxing; promotes a restful sleep
Vapors help open sinus and breathing passages
Lessens pain and helps relieve menstrual discomfort
Increases lactation

Documented Properties

Analgesic, Antiemetic, Antiseptic, Antispasmodic, Aphrodisiac, Aperitive, Calmative, Cardiac, Carminative, Digestive, Disinfectant, Diuretic (*Mild*), Estrogenic, Expectorant, Galactagogue, Hepatic, Insecticide, Laxative, Parasiticide, Pectoral, Stimulant (*Circulatory and Digestive Systems; Respiratory Tract*), Stomachic, Tonic, Warming

Aromatherapy Methods of Use: Application, aroma lamp, bath, inhaler, light bulb ring, massage, mist spray, steam inhalation, steam and sauna room

CAUTION: **Due to the toxicity of the oil, use small amounts. Anise oil can irritate the skin and should either be avoided or used with extra care by people who have sensitive skin.**

ANISE (Star)

Botanical Name: *Illicium verum*
Family: *Illiciaceae*

The essential oil is obtained from the dried seeds of the tree.

History and Information

- Anise star is an evergreen tree native to Asia. The tree grows to a height of about 35 feet, and has shiny green leaves, and small yellow flowers that develop into large star-shaped fruits with brown seeds. The fruits can be eaten fresh or dried, but the leaves are poisonous.

- The use of star anise dates back centuries in Chinese medicine.

- In Asia, the seeds and pods are used to flavor foods.

Practical Uses

Improves digestion; soothes the intestines, relieves flatulence and aerophagy
Calming, relaxing; promotes a restful sleep
Vapors helps open the sinus and breathing passages
Lessens pain and helps relieve mentrual discomfort
Increases lactation

Documented Properties

Analgesic, Antiseptic, Antispasmodic, Aphrodisiac, Aperitive, Calmative, Cardiac, Carminative, Digestive, Disinfectant, Diuretic (*Mild*), Estrogenic, Expectorant, Galactagogue, Insecticide, Stimulant (*Circulatory and Digestive Systems; Respiratory Tract*), Stomachic, Tonic, Warming

Aromatherapy Methods of Use: Application, aroma lamp, bath, inhaler, light bulb ring, massage, mist spray, steam inhalation, steam and sauna room

CAUTION: Due to the toxicity of the oil, use small amounts. Star anise oil can irritate the skin and should either be avoided or used with extra care by people who have sensitive skin.

BASIL (Sweet)

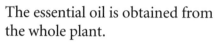

Botanical Name: *Ocimum basilicum*
Family: *Lamiaceae*

The essential oil is obtained from the whole plant.

History and Information

- Sweet basil is a bushy plant native to Africa and Asia. The plant grows to a height of about 2 feet, and has white, blue, or purple flowers. There are approximately 150 different varieties of basil.

- Wreaths of basil have been found in the burial chambers of the ancient Egyptian pyramids.

- Kings were anointed with basil oil during ancient times.

- In Italy, basil symbolizes love. Traditionally, women put a pot of basil outside their window when they are ready for romance.

- The herb is especially known in Asia for its ability to draw out the venomous poisons of a snake or insect bite, when applied directly on the skin.

- In South America and Africa, basil is used for intestinal parasites.

- In China, the herb is used for stomach problems.

- In India, the Hindus consider basil the most sacred of all plants. They plant the herb around their temples, graves, and homes. In Ayurvedic medicine, the plant is used for snakebites, skin problems, and as a tonic.

- In Arabic countries, a tea made from basil is used for menstrual cramps.

Practical Uses

Cooling
Improves digestion
Purifying; helps in the reduction of cellulite
Calming; reduces stress, promotes a restful sleep
Mood uplifting; improves mental clarity and memory, sharpens the senses; helps one to dream; helpful for meditation
Lessens pain
Increases lactation
Neutralizes toxins from insect bites
Soothes insect bites

Documented Properties

Abortifacient, Analgesic, Antibacterial, Antidepressant, Antiseptic, Antispasmodic, Antistress, Antivenomous, Aperitive, Aphrodisiac, Blood Purifier, Carminative, Cephalic, Diaphoretic, Digestive, Emmenagogue, Estrogenic, Expectorant, Febrifuge, Galactagogue, Insect Repellent, Insecticide, Laxative, Nervine, Refreshing, Restorative, Sedative, Stimulant (*Adrenal Glands; Facilitates Childbirth*), Stomachic, Sudorific, Tonic (*Nerves*), Uplifting, Vermifuge

Aromatherapy Methods of Use: Application, aroma lamp, diffusor, inhaler, light bulb ring, massage, mist spray

CAUTION: Due to the toxicity of the oil, use small amounts. Basil oil can irritate the skin and should either be avoided or used with extra care by people who have sensitive skin.

BAY (Sweet)

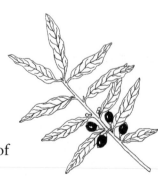

Botanical Name: *Laurus nobilis*
Family: *Lauraceae*

The essential oil is obtained from the leaves of the tree.

History and Information

- Sweet bay is an evergreen tree native to the Mediterranean area, Europe, and the United States. The tree grows to a height of about

10–60 feet, and has green waxy aromatic leaves and small yellow flowers that develop into small black or purple berries.

- In the early Greek and Roman times, bay was the symbol of glory and reward. The greatest honor was bestowed on those fortunate enough to be crowned with the bay laurel wreath. The recipients of the crownings were kings, priests, prophets, poets, scholars, victorious athletes, and soldiers. The Roman generals crowned themselves with bay leaves when they returned home victorious from battle. The soldiers added the leaves to their baths to soothe fatigue and injuries.

- The Romans and Greeks used bay for its valuable memory-improvement property.

- Dioscorides, the Greek physician, used the leaves for insect stings, inflammation, and bladder problems. Galen, the Greek physician, used bay leaves and berries for a variety of ailments, particularly for painful joints and promoting menstruation.

- In the Middle Ages, herbalists used bay to promote menstruation and induce abortions.

- During outbreaks of the plague in Rome, people were advised to live in the vicinity of bay trees.

- During Elizabethan times the leaves were strewn on the floors of homes to freshen stale air.

- Sweet bay oil is also known as laurel leaf oil.

Practical Uses

Warming; improves circulation
Digestive stimulant
Purifying; helps in the reduction of cellulite
Calming; reduces stress
Vapors open sinus and breathing passages
Improves mental clarity and alertness, sharpens the senses
Relieves aching limbs and muscles, lessens pain; good for sprains
Promotes perspiration
Disinfectant
Repels insects

Documented Properties

Analgesic, Antibacterial, Anticoagulant, Antifungal, Antineuralgic, Antipruritic, Antirheumatic, Antiseptic, Antispasmodic, Aperient, Aperitif, Astringent, Carminative, Cholagogue, Diaphoretic, Digestive, Diuretic, Emetic, Emmenagogue, Expectorant, Febrifuge, Hepatic, Hypotensor, Insect Repellent, Nervine, Stimulant (*Digestion*), Stomachic, Tonic

Aromatherapy Methods of Use: Application, aroma lamp, diffusor, inhaler, light bulb ring, massage, mist spray, steam inhalation

CAUTION: Bay oil can irritate the skin and should either be avoided or used with extra care by people who have sensitive skin. Use small amounts.

BAY (West Indian)

Botanical Name: *Myrcia acris, Pimenta acris, P. racemosa*
Family: *Myrtaceae*

The essential oil is obtained from the leaves of the tree.

History and Information

- West Indian bay is a tropical evergreen tree native to the West Indies. It grows to a height of about 30–50 feet, and has aromatic leathery leaves and clusters of white or pink flowers that develop into black oval berries.

- During Victorian times, men used bay rum as a hair dressing. Over the years, bay has been used as a remedy for hair loss and to fragrance colognes and aftershave lotions.

- West Indian bay oil is also known as myrica oil or bay rum oil. It is an ingredient in foods and soft drinks.

Practical Uses

Warming; improves circulation
Digestive stimulant
Purifying; helps in the reduction of cellulite
Calming; reduces stress

Vapors open sinus and breathing passages
Improves mental clarity and alertness, sharpens the senses
Relieves aching limbs and muscles, lessens pain; good for sprains
Promotes perspiration
Disinfectant
Repels insects

Documented Properties

Analgesic, Anticonvulsive, Antifungal, Antineuralgic, Antirheumatic, Antiseptic, Antiviral, Astringent, Expectorant, Hypertensor, Parasiticide, Stimulant, Tonic

Aromatherapy Methods of Use: Application, aroma lamp, diffusor, inhaler, light bulb ring, massage, mist spray, steam inhalation

CAUTION: Bay oil can irritate the skin and should either be avoided or used with extra care by people who have sensitive skin. Use small amounts.

BENZOIN

Botanical Name: *Styrax benzoin, S. tonkinensis*
Family: *Styracaceae*

The resin/essential oil is obtained from the bark of the tree.

History and Information

- Benzoin is native to Asia. The tree grows to a maximum height of 115 feet and has fragrant white flowers. The trunk secretes an aromatic resin when injured. The tree is also known as benjamin tree while the resin is also known as gum benjamin.

- The incense of benzoin has been used for thousands of years in temples during religious ceremonies.

- In France, the resin was burned and inhaled for respiratory problems.

- In southern Asia, benzoin was traditionally used for its healing qualities to mend the wound made by circumcision.

- Benzoin is a common ingredient in skin protective products and cosmetic preparations. It is also used as a preservative in ointments for extending their shelf-life, and a fixative in soaps, perfumes, and creams. The food industry uses benzoin to flavor foods and beverages.

Practical Uses

Warming; improves circulation
Purifying; helps in the reduction of cellulite
Calming; reduces stress, promotes a restful sleep
Improves the breathing and is especially helpful when rubbed on the chest
Mood uplifting; helps one to dream; helpful for meditation
Reduces inflammation, relaxes tight muscles
Acts as a preservative in cosmetics; used as a fixative to hold the scent of a fragrance
Healing to the skin

Documented Properties

Antidepressant, Anti-inflammatory, Antioxidant, Antipruritic, Antiseptic, Antistress, Antitussive, Astringent, Carminative, Cephalic, Cicatrizant, Cordial, Deodorant, Diuretic, Drying, Euphoriant, Expectorant, Fixative, Healing (*Skin*), Pectoral, Preservative, Regulator, Rejuvenator, Sedative, Soothing, Stimulant (*Circulatory System*), Tonic, Uplifting, Vulnerary

Aromatherapy Methods of Use: Application, massage, mist spray

CAUTION: Benzoin resin can irritate the skin and should either be avoided or used with extra care by people who have sensitive skin.

BERGAMOT

Botanical Name: *Citrus bergamia*
Family: *Rutaceae*

The essential oil is made from the peel of the fruit of the tree.

History and Information

- Bergamot is an evergreen citrus tree native to Asia. The tree grows to a height of about 15 feet and bears green to yellow fruit. Bergamot was first discovered growing in Calabria, Italy, in the 17th century. The essence was first sold in the city of Bergamo in the Lombardy region of Italy.

- In Italian folk medicine, the oil was used as a remedy for worms and fevers.

- Bergamot is renowned for its fragrant scent and is widely used in perfumery. The oil is produced from the rind of a fruit similar to the bitter orange. The bergamot fruit should not be confused with an herb in the mint family, monarda, which is also known as bergamot.

Practical Uses

Cooling
Purifying; helps in the reduction of cellulite
Balancing; calming, relieves anxiety, nervous tension and stress; promotes a restful sleep
Mood uplifting, refreshing, improves mental clarity, alertness, sharpens the senses
Disinfectant

Documented Properties

Analgesic, Anthelmintic, Antidepressant, Antiseptic, Antispasmodic, Antistress, Antitoxic, Aperitive, Calmative, Carminative, Cicatrizant, Cordial, Deodorant, Digestive, Expectorant, Febrifuge, Insecticide, Laxative, Parasiticide, Refreshing, Rubefacient, Sedative, Stomachic, Tonic, Uplifting, Vermifuge, Vulnerary

Aromatherapy Methods of Use: Application, aroma lamp, bath, diffusor, inhaler, light bulb ring, massage, mist spray

CAUTION: Bergamot oil can irritate the skin and should either be avoided or used with extra care by people who have sensitive skin. Bergamot is phototoxic. Avoid exposure to direct sunlight several hours after applying the oil on the skin.

BIRCH (Sweet)

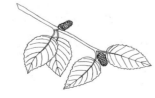

Botanical Name: *Betula capinefolia, B. lenta*
Family: *Betulaceae*

The essential oil is obtained from the tree bark.

History and Information

- Sweet birch is native to North America. The tree grows to a height of about 50–80 feet. The bark is black and the leaves smell of wintergreen. The tree is also known as black birch.

- The American Indians used the birch leaves and dried bark as a tea to relieve headaches, rheumatism, painful menstruation, and abdominal cramps. The essential oil, distilled from the bark, was used for rheumatism, gout, bladder infection, neuralgia, inflammation, and pain. The tree sap was used as a syrup.

- Sweet birch oil was in great demand during the 19th century. As a result, the population of birch trees was decimated, only to recover when wintergreen oil began to be produced synthetically.

- The Russian people have used birch leaves in steam baths throughout history.

- Birch bark is used in medicated soaps to treat skin infections and blemishes; the wood is used to make canoes; and the branches are used for birch beer.

- The sweet birch tree and wintergreen plant produce an oil that is closely identical in smell and chemical composition, but sweet birch yields a greater amount of oil.

Practical Uses

Warming; improves circulation
Purifying; helps in the reduction of cellulite
Calming; relaxes the nerves, reduces tension and stress, promotes a restful sleep
Mood uplifting
Relieves achy, tense, and sore muscles, reduces inflammation; lessens pain, especially in the joints

Documented Properties

Analgesic, Anthelmintic, Anti-inflammatory, Antirheumatic, Antiseptic, Antitoxic, Astringent, Deputative, Detersive, Disinfectant, Diuretic, Febrifuge, Insect Repellent, Insecticide, Laxative, Rubefacient, Stimulant (*Circulatory System*), Tonic

Aromatherapy Methods of Use: Application, aroma lamp, diffusor, inhaler, light bulb ring, massage, mist spray, steam inhalation

CAUTION: Sweet birch is hardly produced anymore and is commonly falsified with the synthetic chemical, methyl salicylate. Due to the toxicity of the "true" oil, use small amounts. Sweet birch can irritate the skin and should either be avoided or used with extra care by people who have sensitive skin.

BIRCH (White)

Botanical Name: *Betula alba*
Family: *Betulaceae*

The essential oil is obtained from the buds and bark of the tree.

History and Information

- White birch is native to the northern hemisphere. The tree grows to a height of about 60 feet.

- Early American settlers used the sap to prevent and treat scurvy, and as a laxative and diuretic.

- The American Indians used the bark and leaves to cleanse and disinfect skin conditions.

- White birch oil has a smoky odor, unlike sweet birch oil. Birch tar is obtained from the bark. The oil extracted from the buds is referred to as birch bud oil and used primarily in shampoos and hair tonics.

Practical Uses

Purifying; helps in the reduction of cellulite
Relieves achy, tense, and sore muscles, reduces inflammation; lessens pain, especially in the joints

Documented Properties

Anti-inflammatory, Antiseptic, Cholagogue, Diaphoretic, Diuretic, Febrifuge, Tonic

Aromatherapy Methods of Use: Application, massage

BOIS de ROSE (Rosewood)

Botanical Name: *Aniba rosaeodora*
Family: *Lauraceae*

The essential oil is obtained from the tree bark.

History and Information

- Bois de rose is an evergreen tree native to the tropical parts of America, the West Indies, and India. It grows to a height of about 80 feet, and has leathery leaves and red flowers. Bois de rose is part of a species of forty evergreen trees.

- Amazonian natives have used the bark for its remarkable property to rejuvenate the skin.

Practical Uses

Calming; relieves nervousness and stress
Mood uplifting
Lessens pain
Regenerates and moisturizes the skin

Documented Properties

Analgesic, Antibacterial, Anticonvulsive, Antidepressant, Antifungal, Antiseptic (*Throat*), Antiviral, Aphrodisiac, Calmative, Cephalic, Deodorant, Emollient (*Skin*), Euphoriant, Insecticide, Parasiticide, Regenerator (*Skin Tissue*), Stimulant (*Immune System*), Tonic, Uplifting

Aromatherapy Methods of Use: Application, aroma lamp, bath, diffusor, inhaler, light bulb ring, massage, mist spray

CABREUVA

Botanical Name: *Myrocarpus fastigiatus*
Family: *Fabaceae*

The essential oil is obtained from the wood chips of the tree.

History and Information

- Cabreuva is native to South America and grows abundantly in forests off the coast of South America. The tree grows to a height of about 50 feet.

- Cabreuva wood is heavy, hard, and durable. It is valued in the production of furniture. The oil is used in fragrances.

Practical Uses

Warming; loosens tight muscles
Calming; reduces stress and tension
Helps to breathe easier
Mood uplifting, aphrodisiac, euphoric; improves mental clarity and alertness
Reduces pain

Documented Properties

Anti-inflammatory, Antiseptic, Aphrodisiac, Balsamic, Cicatrizant, Expectorant, Fixative

Aromatherapy Methods of Use: Application, aroma lamp, bath, diffusor, light bulb ring, inhaler, massage, mist spray

CADE

Botanical Name: *Juniperus oxycedrus*
Family: *Cupressaceae*

The essential oil is obtained from the wood chips and branches of the shrub.

History and Information

- Cade is an evergreen shrub native to the Asian and the Mediterranean region. The shrub grows to a height of about 15–35 feet. Cade is also known as prickly juniper or prickly cedar.

- Through the years, cade oil has been used for snakebites, leprosy, to soothe toothaches, kill lice and their eggs, and heal skin conditions, especially psoriasis.

- Cade is used in perfumery, especially in men's fragrances, and as a food flavoring for a smoky taste. Veterinary practitioners use the oil for parasitic skin problems.

Practical Uses

Relieves aches and pains
Skin care

Documented Properties

Analgesic, Antipruritic, Antiseptic, Disinfectant, Parasiticide (*Skin*), Vermifuge

Aromatherapy Methods of Use: Application, aroma lamp, light bulb ring, massage, mist spray

CAJEPUT

Botanical Name: *Melaleuca cajuputi, M. leucadendron, M. minor*
Family: *Myrtaceae*

The essential oil is obtained from the leaves and buds of the tree.

History and Information

- Cajeput is an evergreen tree native to Australia and Asia. The tree grows to a height of about 50–100 feet and is cultivated in many areas as an ornamental tree for its outstanding white, pink, or purple flowers. Cajeput belongs to a family of over 150 trees.

- In Malaysia and Java, cajeput oil was a traditional remedy for cholera and rheumatism. In Malaysia, the tree is called cajuputi, which means white wood.

- In Africa and Asia, the oil is used an insecticide and parasiticide.

Practical Uses

Slightly warming; improves circulation
Calming, reduces stress; promotes a restful sleep
Vapors open sinus and breathing passages
Relieves aches and pains
Disinfectant
Repels insects

Documented Properties

Analgesic, Anthelmintic, Antibacterial, Antidote, Anti-inflammatory, Antineuralgic, Antipruritic, Antirheumatic, Antiseptic, Antispasmodic, Balsamic, Calmative, Carminative, Cicatrizant, Counter-irritant, Decongestant, Diaphoretic, Emollient (*Skin*), Estrogenic, Expectorant, Febrifuge, Germicide, Healing, Insecticide, Parasiticide, Pectoral, Stimulant (*Circulatory System*), Sudorific, Tonic, Vermifuge

Aromatherapy Methods of Use: Application, aroma lamp, bath, diffusor, inhaler, light bulb ring, massage, mist spray, steam inhalation, steam and sauna room

CALAMINT (Catnip)

Botanical Name: *Calamintha clinopodium, C. grandiflora, C. officinalis, Nepeta cataria, Satureja calamintha*
Family: *Lamiaceae*

The essential oil is obtained from the flowering tops of the plant.

History and Information

- Calamint is a bushy plant native to Europe and Asia. The aromatic plant grows to a height of about 3 feet, and has a flowering spike with small pink flowers and mint-scented leaves.

- Culpeper, the herbalist, found calamint useful for shortness of breath, cramps, and intestinal worms.

- In Europe, a leaf infusion was used for coughs and as a poultice for skin injuries.

- Felines are attracted to and become playful in the presence of calamint.

Practical Uses

Calming
Mood uplifting; improves mental clarity and alertness
Lessens pain

Documented Properties

Analgesic, Antirheumatic, Antispasmodic, Aperitive, Astringent, Carminative, Diaphoretic, Emmenagogue, Expectorant, Febrifuge, Hypnotic, Sedative, Tonic

Aromatherapy Methods of Use: Application, aroma lamp, bath, diffusor, inhaler, light bulb ring, massage, mist spray, steam inhalation, steam and sauna room

CALAMUS (Sweet Flag)

Botanical Name: *Acorus calamus, Calamus aromaticus*
Family: *Araceae*

The essential oil is obtained from the root of the plant.

History and Information

- Calamus is native to Europe, Asia, and North America. The plant grows to a height of about 2–6 feet, and has sword-like leaves and yellow-green flowers.

- The herb has been used for 4000 years.

- The Turkish people use the roots to treat infections. The candied roots are eaten as a preventative against disease and for coughs.

- Asians use the root for its aphrodisiac effect. The Chinese also use calamus to treat deafness, dizziness, and epileptic seizures.

- In India, the powdered herb serves as an insecticide.

- Calamus yields approximately 2% essential oil, which is used in cosmetics, shampoos, perfumes, and as an ingredient in foods and liqueurs. Chewing gum and breath fresheners are produced from the roots.

Documented Properties

Antibacterial, Anticonvulsive, Anti-inflammatory, Antiseptic, Antispasmodic, Aperitive, Aphrodisiac, Carminative, Diaphoretic, Digestive, Expectorant, Febrifuge, Hypotensor, Insect Repellent, Refreshing, Restorative (*Brain; Nervous System*), Sedative, Stimulant (*Salivary Glands*), Stomachic, Tonic, Vermifuge

CAUTION: The calamus that grows in India contains a high content of the component asarone, which is potentially toxic and carcinogenic. However, the plants from North America and Russia do not contain the toxic substance.

CAMPHOR

Botanical Name: *Cinnamomum camphora, Laurus camphora*
Family: *Lauraceae*

The essential oil is obtained from the tree wood.

History and Information

- Camphor is a semi-evergreen tree native to Asia. The tree grows to a maximum height of about 100 feet, and has red leaves that turn green and clusters of yellow flowers. Camphor is related to the cinnamon and cassia trees.

- Camphor has been used in Chinese medicine for 2000 years.

- The price of camphor was once higher than the price of gold.

- Ayurvedic medicine uses the plant for headaches, infections, and snake and insect bites.

Practical Uses

Vapors open sinus and breathing passages
Mood uplifting

Documented Properties

Analgesic, Anthelmintic, Antibacterial, Antidepressant, Anti-inflammatory, Antiseptic, Antispasmodic, Antiviral, Cardiac, Carminative, Counter-irritant, Diuretic, Expectorant, Febrifuge, Hypertensive, Insect Repellent, Insecticide, Laxative, Rubefacient, Sedative, Stimulant (*Central Nervous System; Adrenal Glands; Respiratory System*), Sudorific, Vasoconstrictor, Vermifuge, Vulnerary

CAUTION: Camphor oil is an adrenal stimulant and can be harmful. Avoid if prone to epileptic seizures. Do not use on children.

CAMPHOR (Borneol)

Botanical Name: *Dryobalanops aromatica, D. camphora*
Family: *Dipterocarpaceae*

The essential oil is obtained from the tree wood.

History and Information

- Borneol camphor is a tall evergreen tree native to Asia. The tree grows to about 50–160 feet high, and has leathery leaves and small white flowers.

- Camphor has been highly regarded in Asian countries for over 2000 years. It was used as a remedy against the plagues.

Practical Uses

Vapors open the sinus and breathing passages
Mood uplifting
Adrenal stimulant

Documented Properties

Analgesic, Antidepressant, Anti-inflammatory, Antiseptic, Antispasmodic, Antiviral, Carminative, Diuretic, Rubefacient, Stimulant (*Adrenal Glands*), Tonic

CAUTION: Borneol camphor should only be used in small amounts since it can cause an overstimulation of the adrenal glands. Exercise caution when using this oil.

CANANGA

Botanical Name: *Cananga odorata*
Family: *Annonaceae*

The essential oil is obtained from the tree's flowers.

History and Information

- Cananga is an evergreen tree native to Asia. The tree grows to a height of about 100 feet, and has large yellow fragrant flowers and glossy leaves.

- In the 19th century, cananga was an ingredient in a European hair oil.

Practical Uses

Calming, reduces stress; promotes a restful sleep
Mood uplifting, euphoric
Lessens pain, relaxes the muscles

Documented Properties

Antidepressant, Antiseptic, Aphrodisiac, Emollient, Euphoriant, Fixative, Hypotensor, Nervine, Relaxant, Sedative, Tonic

Aromatherapy Methods of Use: Application, aroma lamp, bath, diffusor, inhaler, light bulb ring, massage, mist spray

CARAWAY

Botanical Name: *Apium carvi, Carum carvi*
Family: *Apiaceae*

The essential oil is obtained from the seeds of the plant.

History and Information

- Caraway is native to Europe and Asia. The plant grows to a height of about 2 feet, and has carrot-like leaves, small white or pink flowers, seed capsules that bursts open when mature, and a fleshy root that looks like a carrot.

- Caraway seeds have been in use for 5000 years. In the Ebers Papyrus in 1550 B.C., the ancient Egyptians recommended caraway for digestive upsets.

- Dioscorides, the Greek physician, suggested eating the seeds to aid digestion.

- Caraway is used to promote menstruation, lactation in nursing mothers, and for menstrual cramps. A cream made from the herb was used by European women to remove wrinkles and beautify their skin.

- Caraway was once an essential ingredient in love potions.

- Country people fed their animals caraway to keep them from straying.

- The seeds yield 3–5% essential oil, which is used to flavor two digestive aid liqueurs, Scandinavian Aquavit and German Kümmel. Caraway seeds are often used in breads, pastries, and sauces to aid the digestive process and relieve flatulence.

Practical Uses

Improves digestion; soothes the intestines, relieves flatulence
Relieves pain and menstrual discomfort

Documented Properties

Abortifacient, Antibacterial, Antiseptic, Antispasmodic, Aperitive, Astringent, Cardiac, Carminative, Depurative, Digestive, Disinfectant, Diuretic, Emmenagogue, Expectorant (*Mild*), Galactagogue, Parasiticide, Regenerator (*Tissue*), Stimulant (*Circulation; Digestive and Glandular Systems*), Stomachic, Tonic (*Nerves and Digestive Organs*), Vermifuge

Aromatherapy Methods of Use: Application, aroma lamp, bath, diffusor, inhaler, light bulb ring, massage, mist spray

CARDAMOM

Botanical Name: *Elettaria cardamomum*
Family: *Zingiberaceae*

The essential oil is obtained from the seeds of the plant.

History and Information

- Cardamom is native to Asia. The plant grows to a height of about 10 feet and has small yellow flowers. The fruit holds eighteen seeds.

- Cardamom was first brought to the West by soldiers of Alexander the Great upon returning from India.

- The earliest reports of Ayurvedic medicine mentioned cardamom for its use in urinary problems and reducing body fat. Cardamom has also been used as a remedy for hemorrhoids, nausea, headaches, and fever.

- The Romans ate the seeds to aid digestion.

- Chinese medicine considers cardamom invaluable for intestinal problems. It is also used for pulmonary diseases and fevers.

- Cardamom is the most popular spice in the Arab countries. A coffee made from the seeds is consumed regularly by the people of Saudi Arabia. In Scandinavian countries, the seeds are used in pastries.

- Approximately 80% of the world's supply of cardamom is produced in India. The fruits and seeds yield approximately 4–7% essential oil.

Practical Uses

Warming; improves circulation
Improves digestion; soothes the intestines, relieves flatulence
Mood uplifting, energizing, improves mental clarity, improves physical strength, increases sexual strength
Relieves pain, menstrual pains and cramps

Documented Properties

Antiseptic, Antispasmodic, Aperitif, Aperitive, Aphrodisiac, Calmative, Carminative, Cephalic, Digestive, Diuretic, Expectorant, Refreshing, Stimulant (*Circulation; Digestion*), Stomachic, Tonic, Uplifting

Aromatherapy Methods of Use: Application, aroma lamp, bath, diffusor, inhaler, light bulb ring, massage, mist spray

CARNATION (Clove Pink)

Botanical Name: *Dianthus caryophyllus*
Family: *Caryophyllaceae*

The absolute/essential oil is obtained from the flowers of the plant.

History and Information

- The carnation plant originated in Europe. The bushy plant reaches a height of about 2 feet. The flowers emit a fragrance that intensifies towards the evening.

- Carnations were the most popular flower used in garlands, chaplets, and coronets at coronation ceremonies; thus, its name was derived from the word "coronation."

- The oil is extracted from the double-flowered variety of clove pink, which has a spicy fragrance.

Practical Uses

Mood uplifting

Documented Properties

Antidepressant, Antistress, Calmative, Sedative

Aromatherapy Methods of Use: Application, aroma lamp, fragrancing, inhaler, light bulb ring, massage, mist spray

CASCARILLA BARK

Botanical Name: *Croton eleuteria*
Family: *Euphorbiaceae*

The essential oil is obtained from the tree bark.

History and Information

- Cascarilla is native to the West Indies and Central America. The tree grows to a height of about 40 feet and has small white fragrant flowers that develop into a seed capsule.

- In Latin America, a stimulating drink is brewed from the leaves and bark.

- In China, the bark is used for malaria, pain, and nausea.

- The bark emits an aromatic scent when burned. Cascarilla is used extensively in cigarettes for their aroma when smoked. The oil is used to fragrance soaps, detergents, cosmetics, perfumes, and as an ingredient to flavor foods and beverages. The yield of essential oil is approximately 2%. An oil is also made from the seeds, but it is dangerous due to the strong purgative effect.

Practical Uses

Warming
Calming; reduces stress and tension
Helps to deepen breathing
Mood uplifting, euphoric

Documented Properties

Antiseptic, Astringent, Carminative, Digestive, Expectorant, Stomachic, Tonic

Aromatherapy Methods of Use: Application, bath, massage, mist spray

CASSIA

Botanical Name: *Cinnamomum aromaticum, C. cassia, Laurus cassia*
Family: *Lauraceae*

The essential oil is obtained from the young leaves and twigs of the tree.

History and Information

- Cassia is an evergreen tree native to Asia. The tree grows to a height of about 80 feet, and has small green flowers and a thin-peeling bark.

- Cassia was considered one of the most important herbs used in the Greek and Roman pharmacopoeia. Cassia leaves were also mentioned as a spice in a 1st century Roman cookbook.

- Its name is derived from the Greek word *kassia*, which means "to strip off the bark." This refers to the way the essential oil is obtained by stripping the bark and boiling it. The bark yields approximately 2% of essential oil. Cassia has a stronger aroma than cinnamon, is cheaper in price, and is sometimes referred to as "poor man's cinnamon."

Practical Uses

Heating; improves circulation
Helps in the reduction of cellulite
Mood uplifting, reviving, helps to relieve a fatigued state
Lessens pain, increases mobility in the joints
Disinfectant
Repels insects

Documented Properties

Analgesic, Antibacterial, Antiemetic, Antifungal, Antiseptic, Antiviral, Aphrodisiac, Astringent, Carminative, Emmenagogue, Laxative, Parasiticide, Stimulant (*Increases Contractions During Childbirth; Circulatory System*), Vasodilator

Aromatherapy Methods of Use: Aroma lamp, diffusor, light bulb ring, mist spray

CAUTION: Because of cassia's heating property, the oil can cause skin irritation on many people. It is not advised to be used for application on the skin.

CASSIE

Botanical Name: *Acacia farnesiana, Cassia ancienne*
Family: *Mimosaceae*

The absolute/essential oil is obtained from the flowers of the bush.

History and Information

- Cassie is native to the West Indies and tropical America. The bush grows to a height of about 5–25 feet, and has leathery leaflets and tiny, sweet fragrant yellow flowers that develop into kidney-shaped seeds in a pod.

- In Central America, a drink from the infused flowers is taken for stomach troubles, headaches, and to calm the nerves.

- In India, cassie is made into a perfume.

- In China, the flowers are used for rheumatism and chest ailments.

- The oil is added to fragrance expensive perfumes and as a food flavoring.

Practical Uses

Mood uplifting

Documented Properties

Antirheumatic, Antiseptic, Antispasmodic, Aphrodisiac, Balsamic, Insecticide

Aromatherapy Methods of Use: Fragrancing

CEDARWOOD

Botanical Name: *Juniperus virginiana*
Family: *Cupressaceae*

The essential oil is obtained from the sawdust and wood chips of the red cedar tree.

History and Information

- Cedarwood is an evergreen tree native to North America. The tree grows to a height of over 100 feet.

- The American Indians burned the twigs and inhaled the smoke to relieve head colds and chest congestion. The fumes were also used to promote childbirth delivery.

- Pencils are made from the wood of the tree.

Practical Uses

Calming; relieves anxiety and nervous tension, promotes a restful sleep
Vapors open the sinus and breathing passages; eases chest congestion when rubbed on the chest
Helps one to dream; helpful for meditation
Lessens pain
Repels insects

Documented Properties

Abortifacient, Antipruritic, Antiseptic, Antispasmodic, Astringent, Balsamic, Diuretic, Emmenagogue, Emollient, Expectorant, Healing (*Skin*), Insect Repellent, Sedative, Stimulant (*Circulatory System*)

Aromatherapy Methods of Use: Application, aroma lamp, bath, inhaler, light bulb ring, massage, mist spray, steam inhalation, steam and sauna room

CAUTION: Due to the toxicity of the oil, use small amounts.

CEDARWOOD (Atlas)

Botanical Name: *Cedrus atlantica*
Family: *Pinaceae*

The essential oil is obtained from the wood of the tree.

History and Information

- Cedarwood is an evergreen tree native to Africa. The tree grows to a height of about 130–140 feet and has needle-like leaves. If undisturbed, the tree can reach an age of 1000 to 2000 years.

- A grove of cedars from which King Solomon built his temple still exists today on Mount Lebanon. The first cedar planted in Great Britain, in 1646, is still living today.

- The wood was thought to be indestructible and, therefore, was used in the building of King Solomon's temple in Jerusalem. It also had been used to build palaces, mummy cases, and furniture.

- Cedarwood was highly prized and valued by the Egyptians for its use in cosmetics. It was also burned in the temples of Egypt and Greece.

- The oil is used extensively in hair and skin care products. In France, it is added to shampoos and lotions to protect the hair and prevent hair loss.

Practical Uses

Cooling
Calming; relieves anxiety and nervous tension, promotes a restful sleep
Vapors open the sinus and breathing passages; eases chest congestion when rubbed on the chest
Improves mental clarity
Helps one to dream; helpful for meditation
Lessens pain, loosens tight muscles
Repels insects

Documented Properties

Antidepressant, Antifungal, Antiputrid, Antiseptic, Aphrodisiac, Astringent, Detoxifier (*Cellulite*), Diuretic, Expectorant, Fixative, Insect Repellent, Regenerator (*Skin*), Sedative, Stimulant (*Circulatory System*), Tonic

Aromatherapy Methods of Use: Application, aroma lamp, bath, inhaler, light bulb ring, massage, mist spray, steam inhalation, steam and sauna room

CELERY

Botanical Name: *Apium graveolens*
Family: *Apiaceae*

The essential oil is obtained from the seeds of the plant.

History and Information

- Celery is native to the Mediterranean area. The plant grows to a height of about 1–2 feet and has white flowers.

- The Romans and Greeks grew celery for medicinal values. The Greeks also made a celery wine, which was given to victorious athletes.

- Ayurvedic physicians in India have used celery seeds since ancient times for water retention, joint problems, and indigestion.

- In Europe, the seeds are a common medicinal treatment for gout and rheumatism.

- The seeds yield approximately 2% essential oil. Celery oil is an ingredient in foods, liqueurs, perfumes, and soaps.

Practical Uses

Cooling
Purifying; helps in the reduction of cellulite
Promotes a calm, relaxed state and a restful sleep

Documented Properties

Abortifacient, Analgesic, Antiarthritic, Anticonvulsive, Antilithic, Antioxidant, Antiphlogistic, Antirheumatic, Antiscorbutic, Antispasmodic, Aperitive, Aphrodisiac, Carminative, Cholagogue, Depurative, Diaphoretic, Digestive, Diuretic, Emmenagogue, Hepatic, Hypotensor, Nervine, Sedative, Stimulant (*Uterine Contractions*), Stomachic, Tonic, Vulnerary

Aromatherapy Methods of Use: Application, aroma lamp, bath, inhaler, light bulb ring, massage, mist spray

CAUTION: Because of celery's detoxifying effect, use small amounts.

CHAMOMILE (German) & CHAMOMILE (Roman)

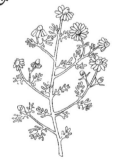

Botanical Name: *Matricaria chamomilla, M. recutica* (German chamomile); *Anthemis nobilis, Chamaemelum nobile* (Roman chamomile)
Family: *Asteraceae*

The essential oil is obtained from the flowers and leaves of the plant.

History and Information

- German chamomile is native to Europe and Asia. The plant grows to a height of about 3 feet and has small daisy-like yellow flowerheads with white petals.

- Roman chamomile is native to Europe and Asia. The plant grows to a height of about 1 foot and has flowers that are similar in appearance to daisies.

- Dioscorides and Galen, Greek physicians, used chamomile for female ailments and fevers. In southern Europe, chamomile is still used for childbearing and female problems.

- The Egyptian sages dedicated the plant to the sun for its ability to reduce fevers. The flowers were powdered and used to relieve pain.

- Chamomile is one of the most popular herbal teas in the Western world.

- Chamomile contains a component called azulene, which is formed after the essential oil is distilled. The German variety yields a greater amount. Azulene has been found to be an excellent anti-inflammatory agent.

Practical Uses

Improves digestion; soothes the intestines
Calming, promotes a restful sleep
Mood uplifting
Lessens pain, relieves menstrual discomfort, soothes inflammation
Healing to the skin; soothes insect bites

Documented Properties

Analgesic, Antianemic, Antibacterial, Anticonvulsive, Antidepressant, Antiemetic, Antifungal, Anti-inflammatory, Antineuralgic, Antipruritic, Antirheumatic, Antiseptic, Antispasmodic, Antistress, Antitoxic, Aperitive, Calmative, Carminative, Cholagogue, Cicatrizant, Digestive, Diuretic, Emmenagogue, Emollient, Febrifuge, Healing, Hepatic, Hypotensor, Laxative, Nervine, Regenerator (*Skin*), Sedative, Stimulant (*Digestive System; Spleen, Uterine*), Stomachic, Sudorific, Tonic, Vermifuge, Vulnerary

Aromatherapy Methods of Use: Application, aroma lamp, bath, diffusor, inhaler, light bulb ring, massage, mist spray

CHAMOMILE (Moroccan)

Botanical Name: *Anthemis mixta, Ormenis mixta, O. multicaulis*
Family: *Asteraceae*

The essential oil is obtained from the flowering tops of the plant.

History and Information

● Moroccan chamomile is native to Africa and the Mediterranean area.

Practical Uses

Calming

Documented Properties

Anti-inflammatory, Antiseptic, Antispasmodic, Calmative, Cholagogue, Emmenagogue, Hepatic, Parasiticide, Sedative, Tonic

Aromatherapy Methods of Use: Application, aroma lamp, bath, diffusor, inhaler, light bulb ring, massage, mist spray

CHAMPACA FLOWER & LEAF

Botanical Name: *Michelia alba, M. champaca*
Family: *Magnoliaceae*

The champaca flower essential oil is obtained from the flowers. The champaca leaf essential oil is obtained from the leaves of the tree.

History and Information

● Champaca is an evergreen tree native to Asia. The tree grows to a height of about 65 feet, and has long glossy leaves and small fragrant white flowers.

● The tree is planted in India around temples to supply flowers for religious ceremonies.

● In India, the bark of the tree is used as a remedy to reduce fever and the roots are used for skin disorders.

● Champaca is also known as frangipani.

Practical Uses for the Flower Oil

Warming
Calming, promotes a peaceful state; reduces stress
Helps to breathe easier
Mood uplifting, euphoric

Practical Uses for the Leaf Oil

Warming
Calming; reduces stress
Helps to breathe easier
Euphoric; improves mental clarity

Documented Properties

Aphrodisiac, Emollient, Febrifuge

Aromatherapy Methods of Uses: Application, aroma lamp, bath, fragrancing, inhaler, light bulb ring, massage, mist spray

CINNAMON BARK & LEAF

Botanical Name: *Cinnamomum verum, C. zeylanicum, Laurus cinnamomum*
Family: *Lauraceae*

The essential oil of cinnamon bark is obtained from the bark of the tree. The essential oil of cinnamon leaf is obtained from the leaves of the tree.

History and Information

● Cinnamon is an evergreen tree native to Asia. The tree grows to a height of about 50 feet, and has leathery leaves and small white flowers that develop into light blue berries.

● Cinnamon is one of the oldest spices mentioned in the Old Testament. Chinese herbalists wrote about cinnamon as early as 2700 B.C. and used it for fever, diarrhea, and menstrual problems.

● The cinnamon tree has been cultivated in Ceylon since 1200 A.D.

- The Egyptians used cinnamon in their embalming procedures.

- The Greek and Roman pharmacopoeia recognized cinnamon as one of the most important herbs for its strong antiseptic properties.

- Cinnamon was one of the most sought-after spices in the explorations of the 15th and 16th centuries. At one time, the spice was more valuable than gold.

- In Chinese medicine, many herbal remedies require the inclusion of cinnamon. Some of the uses include a tonic for depression, a calmative, and a strengthener for the heart.

- Studies by Japanese researchers have shown that cinnamon kills fungi, bacteria, and other microorganisms, including the bacteria responsible for botulism poisoning and staph infections.

- The bark yields 0.5–1.5% essential oil, which becomes darker when it is exposed to air.

Practical Uses

Heating; improves circulation
Improves digestion
Purifying; helps in the reduction of cellulite
Reduces stress
Mood uplifting, reviving, helps to relieve a fatigued state
Lessens pain, loosens tight muscles
Disinfectant
Repels insects

Documented Properties

Analgesic, Anesthetic, Anthelmintic, Antibacterial, Antidepressant, Antidiarrhea, Antidote, Antiemetic, Antiputrid, Antirheumatic, Antiseptic (*Strong*), Antispasmodic, Antiviral, Aperitif, Aphrodisiac, Astringent (*Mild*), Antitussive, Cardiac, Carminative, Digestive, Emmenagogue, Febrifuge, Hemostatic, Insecticide, Parasiticide, Stimulant (*Circulatory, Glandular, Nervous, and Respiratory System; Production of Secretions: Saliva, Tears, and Mucous; Uterine Contractions*), Stomachic, Tonic, Vermifuge

Aromatherapy Methods of Use for Cinnamon Bark: Aroma lamp, diffusor, inhaler, light bulb ring, mist spray

Aromatherapy Method of Use for Cinnamon Leaf: Application, aroma lamp, diffusor, inhaler, light bulb ring, massage, mist spray

CAUTION: Cinnamon bark should not be used on the skin. Cinnamon leaf oil can irritate the skin and should either be avoided or used with extra care by people who have sensitive skin.

CITRONELLA

Botanical Name: *Andropogon nardus, Cymbopogon nardus*
Family: *Poaceae*

The essential oil is obtained from the grass.

History and Information

- Citronella is an aromatic tall grass native to Asia.

- Citronella is also known as mana grass and is widely used in soaps, perfumery, and sanitary products. Since the oil is inexpensive, it is used to adulterate other essential oils such as rose oil.

Practical Uses

Cooling
Calming, reduces stress
Mood uplifting; mental stimulant, improves mental clarity and alertness
Repels insects

Documented Properties

Antibacterial, Antidepressant, Antifungal, Anti-inflammatory, Antiseptic, Antispasmodic, Deodorant, Deodorizer, Diaphoretic, Disinfectant, Diuretic, Emmenagogue, Febrifuge, Insect Repellent, Insecticide, Parasiticide, Stimulant (*Digestion*), Stomachic, Tonic, Uplifting, Vermifuge

Aromatherapy Methods of Use: Application, aroma lamp, diffusor, inhaler, light bulb ring, massage, mist spray

CAUTION: Citronella oil can irritate the skin and should either be avoided or used with extra care by people who have sensitive skin. Citronella is phototoxic. Avoid exposure to direct sunlight several hours after applying the oil on the skin.

CLARY SAGE

Botanical Name: *Salvia sclarea*
Family: *Lamiaceae*

The essential oil is obtained from the flowering tops of the plant.

History and Information

- Clary sage is native to Europe. The plant grows to a height of about 3 feet, and has flowers that are pink, white, or blue, depending on the variety.

- In the 1500's, clary sage was cultivated in Europe mainly for brewing ales and adding to wine to make it more intoxicating.

- Clary sage is known to contain a hormone similar to the one produced by females. It is useful in helping women with sexual problems, menstrual discomfort, and premenstrual tension.

Practical Uses

Improves digestion
Calming; relieves stress and tension, promotes a restful sleep
Mood uplifting; aphrodisiac, increases sexual strength
Relieves menstrual pain and cramps; regulates the female reproductive system

Documented Properties

Analgesic, Anticonvulsive, Antidepressant, Anti-inflammatory, Antiseptic, Antispasmodic, Antistress, Antisudorific, Aphrodisiac, Astringent, Balsamic, Calmative, Carminative, Deodorant, Digestive, Emmenagogue, Emollient, Estrogenic, Euphoriant, Fixative, Healing (*Skin*), Hypotensor, Nervine, Refreshing, Relaxant (*Strong*), Regenerator (*Skin Cells*), Sedative, Stimulant (*Uterine Contractions*), Stomachic, Tonic, Tonifying, Uplifting, Warming

Aromatherapy Methods of Use: Application, aroma lamp, bath, diffusor, inhaler, light bulb ring, massage, mist spray

CAUTION: Due to the relaxing effect of the oil, clary sage should not be used before driving or doing anything that requires full attention. In large amounts, clary sage can be stupefying on the mind. Use small amounts at a time.

CLOVE BUD, LEAF & STEM

Botanical Name: *Eugenia aromatica, E. caryophyllata, E. caryophyllus, Syzygium aromaticum*
Family: *Myrtaceae*

Clove bud essential oil is obtained from the buds of the tree. Clove leaf essential oil is obtained from the leaves. Clove stem essential oil is obtained from the stems.

History and Information

- Clove is an tropical evergreen tree native to Asia. The tree grows to a height of about 40 feet, and has dark green leaves and bright pink buds that develop first into yellow flowers, then into purple berries.

- In ancient Persia, clove was used in love potions.

- In Chinese medicine, clove is known for its antibacterial and antifungal properties.

- Ayurvedic healers in India have used clove to treat fevers and respiratory and digestive ailments.

- The people of the Molucca Islands were devastated by previously unknown epidemics after the Dutch destroyed all the clove trees.

- A folk remedy for the relief of headaches consisted of clove and apple-cider vinegar.

- Folk healers, pharmacists, and dentists have prescribed cloves, or clove oil, to relieve toothaches.

- Clove oil was used to disinfect large public places like theatres.

- The buds yield 16% essential oil, the stems 4–6%, and the leaves 2%. The oils are used in perfumes, soaps, toothpastes, and mouthwashes. It is reported that Indonesian people consume almost 65% of the world's supply of cloves to make their own cigarettes by mixing it with tobacco.

Practical Uses

Heating
Improves digestion; relieves flatulence
Vapors open sinus and breathing passages
Mood uplifting, reviving, aphrodisiac; mental stimulant, improves mental clarity and memory
Reduces pain by numbing the area
Disinfectant
Repels insects

Documented Properties

Abortifacient, Analgesic, Anesthetic (*Local*), Anthelmintic, Antibacterial, Antidepressant, Antiemetic, Antifungal, Antineuralgic, Antioxidant, Antirheumatic, Antiseptic (*Strong*), Antispasmodic, Antistress, Antiviral, Aperitif, Aphrodisiac, Carminative, Caustic, Cicatrizant, Counter-irritant, Disinfectant, Expectorant, Insect Repellent, Insecticide, Parasiticide, Stimulant (*Vitality*), Stomachic, Tonic, Vermifuge

Aromatherapy Methods of Use: Application, aroma lamp, diffusor, inhaler, light bulb ring, massage, mist spray

CAUTION: Clove oil can irritate the skin and should either be avoided or used with extra care by people who have sensitive skin. Use small amounts. The oil from clove bud is the only clove oil suitable for use in aromatherapy, since it is less irritating than the leaf and stem oils.

COFFEE

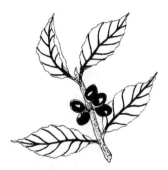

Botanical Name: *Coffea arabica*
Family: *Rubiaceae*

The essential oil is obtained from the beans of the tree.

History and Information

- Coffee is a tropical evergreen tree native to Ethiopia. The tree has glossy leaves and small white flowers with a jasmine-like fragrance. The flowers develop into sweet-tasting berries with two beans inside. In the wild, the tree grows to a height of about 26–33 feet. When cultivated, it only reaches 14–20 feet, but the trees are usually pruned to 4–6 feet. There are more than twenty-five species of the coffee tree.

- Prior to being made into a hot beverage drink, coffee was used as a food, wine, and medicine.

- The Muslims highly prized coffee and drank it during prayers, even in the Holy Temple in Mecca.

- By the 13th century, coffee became a mainstay of Arabian life. Coffee houses emerged everywhere and became a meeting place where people gathered to discuss events of the day. Until the end of the 17th century, practically all coffee was produced in Arabia.

- Coffee drinking was condemned by the clergymen of the church until the 17th century, when Pope Clement VIII enjoyed the taste of it so much that he sanctioned its use for all his followers. After his approval, coffee gained in popularity and coffee houses thrived in Europe.

- In Turkey, a wife could once be legally granted a divorce if her husband failed to furnish her with the daily allotment of coffee.

- Coffee is the world's favorite beverage. The United States consumes about 20% of all coffee grown. Brazil is the largest grower of coffee and produces about 25% of the world's supply.

Practical Uses

Warming
Increases appetite
Stimulant
Mood uplifting, energizing; improves mental clarity

Documented Properties

Diuretic, Stimulant

Aromatherapy Methods of Use: Application, aroma lamp, bath, light bulb ring, massage, mist spray

CAUTION: Coffee oil is an adrenal gland and nervous system stimulant. It can be deleterious to a person's health in large amounts.

COPAIBA

Botanical Name: *Copaifera officinalis*
Family: *Fabaceae*

The resin/essential oil is obtained from the tree.

History and Information

- Copaiba is an evergreen tree native to tropical America and Africa. The tree grows to a height of about 60 feet and has small yellow flowers that turn from brown to red fruits. Copaiba is part of a species of about forty evergreen trees.

- The resin is extracted by drilling holes in the tree trunk; one tree can yield up to 12 gallons.

- In Brazil, copaiba sap is made into an ointment to heal the skin.

Practical Uses

Warming; improves circulation
Soothes the intestines
Calming, promotes a peaceful state of mind, reduces stress; promotes a restful sleep
Opens breathing passages; allows deeper breathing
Mood uplifting; improves mental clarity and alertness; helpful for meditation
Used as a fixative to hold the scent of a fragrance
Healing and moisturizing to the skin

Documented Properties

Anthelmintic, Antibacterial, Balsamic, Disinfectant, Diuretic, Expectorant, Stimulant

Aromatherapy Methods of Use: Application, aroma lamp, bath, diffusor, inhaler, light bulb ring, massage, mist spray, steam inhalation, steam and sauna room

CORIANDER

Botanical Name: *Coriandrum sativum*
Family: *Apiaceae*

The essential oil is obtained from the seeds of the ripe fruits and the leaves of the plant.

History and Information

- Coriander is native to the Mediterranean area. The plant grows to a height of about 3 feet and has small white flowers that develop into green seeds. Coriander is also known as cilantro and Chinese parsley.

- The use of coriander dates back to 5000 B.C.

- The Chinese used coriander as far back as the third century B.C. They believed the seeds contained the power of immortality.

- In Ayurvedic medicine, coriander was used to relieve constipation and help sleep.

- Greek and Roman physicians, including Hippocrates, made medicines with coriander. It was also highly prized as a spice, and used as an ingredient in Roman vinegar to preserve meat and flavor bread.

- The Egyptians added coriander seeds to wine to increase the intoxication.

- In the Middle East and Europe, coriander has been valued as a love potion and aphrodisiac.

- To ease the pain and facilitate childbirth, a preparation of coriander seeds was placed on a woman's thighs while she was in labor.

- In European cultures, a tea or soup made from the leaves and mixed with barley water is taken to help a person, who is recovering from an illness, regain strength. In China, coriander seeds are used to break up phlegm, stop bleeding, and for hemorrhoids. The herb is used for indigestion, nausea, and constipation.

- Coriander was listed in the United States pharmacopoeia from 1820 to 1980.

- The seeds yield 0.5–1% essential oil. The oil is used as an ingredient in perfumes, candy, chocolate, baked goods, brewing, many liqueurs, and to flavor beer.

Practical Uses

Improves digestion; relieves flatulence, aerophagy and nausea; strengthens and tones the stomach
Reviving, energizing; improves mental clarity and memory; helps to relieve a fatigued state
Relieves pain

Documented Properties

Abortifacient, Analgesic, Antibacterial, Antioxidant, Antirheumatic, Antispasmodic, Aperitif, Aperitive, Aphrodisiac, Calmative, Carminative, Deodorant, Depurative, Detoxifier, Diaphoretic, Digestive, Diuretic, Nervine, Refreshing, Regenerator, Revitalizing, Stimulant (*Circulatory System*), Stomachic, Tonic, Uplifting, Warming

Aromatherapy Methods of Use: Application, aroma lamp, bath, diffusor, inhaler, light bulb ring, massage, mist spray

CAUTION: Due to the toxicity of the oil, use small amounts.

CORNMINT

Botanical Name: *Mentha arvensis*
Family: *Lamiaceae*

The essential oil is obtained from the plant leaves.

History and Information

- Cornmint is native to North America and Asia. The plant grows to a height of about 1–3 feet, and has aromatic leaves and small clusters of white or purplish flowers.

- The leaves yield an oil that is comprised of approximately 85% menthol. The oil is dementholized because the high menthol content causes it to solidify at room temperature. A large portion of the world's supply of menthol is derived from the cornmint plant.

Practical Uses

Cooling
Improves digestion; relieves flatulence

Vapors open sinus and breathing passages
Mood uplifting especially to people who have a slow metabolism; refreshing, reviving, energizing; improves mental clarity and alertness, sharpens the senses
Lessens pain
Repels insects

Documented Properties

Antibacterial, Antiseptic, Antispasmodic, Carminative, Digestive, Expectorant, Refreshing, Refrigerant, Stimulant, Stomachic

Aromatherapy Methods of Use: Aroma lamp, diffusor, fragrancing, inhaler, light bulb ring, mist spray, steam inhalation, sauna and steam room

COMMENTS: For applications other than fragrancing, use peppermint or spearmint oil, since cornmint is a fractionated oil.

CAUTION: Cornmint oil can irritate the skin and should either be avoided or used with extra care by people who have sensitive skin. Use small amounts. Avoid using before bedtime since the oil can overstimulate the nervous system.

COSTUS

Botanical Name: *Saussurea costus, S. lappa*
Family: *Asteraceae*

The essential oil is obtained from the roots of the plant.

History and Information

- Costus is native to India. The plant grows to a height of about 8 feet.

- Costus root has been used for centuries in Asia as a remedy for cholera, typhoid, and infections.

- In Ayurvedic medicine, costus is used to help rheumatism, asthma, digestive problems, and coughs, and to heal the skin.

- The oil is used to scent perfumes and as a food flavoring.

Practical Uses

Cooling
Calming; promotes a restful sleep
Improves alertness

Documented Properties

Antibacterial, Antiseptic, Antispasmodic, Antiviral, Carminative, Digestive, Expectorant, Febrifuge, Hypotensor, Stimulant, Stomachic, Tonic, Vasodilator

Aromatherapy Methods of Use: Application, aroma lamp, fragrancing, light bulb ring, massage, mist spray

CUBEB

Botanical Name: *Cubeba officinalis, Piper cubeba*
Family: *Piperaceae*

The essential oil is obtained from the berries of the shrub.

History and Information

- Cubeb is an evergreen, climbing woody shrub native to Indonesia. The plant grows to a height of about 20 feet and has clusters of flowers that develop into small berries, which resemble peppers.

- In the 19th century, the dried berries were rolled up into cigarettes and smoked to relieve asthma and chest congestion.

- Cubeb is used as a spice in Europe and Asia.

Practical Uses

Improves circulation
Improves digestion
Vapors open sinus and breathing passages
Relieves aches, pains, and inflammation

Documented Properties

Antibacterial, Anti-inflammatory, Antiseptic (*Strong*), Antispasmodic, Antiviral, Carminative, Diuretic, Expectorant, Stimulant (*Circulatory System*), Stomachic, Tonic

Aromatherapy Methods of Use: Application, aroma lamp, bath, diffusor, inhaler, light bulb ring, massage, mist spray, steam inhalation, steam and sauna room

CUMIN

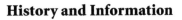

Botanical Name: *Cuminum cyminum, C. odorum*
Family: *Apiaceae*

The essential oil is obtained from the seeds and fruit of the plant.

History and Information

- Cumin is native to the Mediterranean area. The plant grows to height of about 1 foot, has thread-like leaves, small white or pink flowers, and aromatic seeds.

- Cumin has been an ingredient in perfumes, love potions, and baths for its aphrodisiac effect.

- In Ayurvedic medicine, cumin has been used to aid digestion and strengthen convalescing patients.

- Cumin is a spice in Arab, European, and Vietnamese cuisines. It is also used as an ingredient in Indian curry.

- The seeds yield 2–4% essential oil.

Practical Uses

Warming; improves circulation
Improves digestion; relieves flatulence
Purifying; helps in the reduction of cellulite
Calming, reduces stress
Mood uplifting, euphoric; reviving, helps to relieve fatigue; helpful for meditation
Relieves pain

Documented Properties

Analgesic, Antibacterial, Anti-inflammatory, Antioxidant, Antiseptic, Antispasmodic, Antitoxic, Aperitive, Aphrodisiac, Cardiac, Carminative, Depurative, Digestive, Diuretic, Emmenagogue,

Larvicide, Nervine, Parasiticide, Revitalizing, Sedative, Stimulant (*Circulatory, Digestive, and Nervous Systems*), Tonic

Aromatherapy Methods of Use: Application, aroma lamp, diffusor, light bulb ring, massage, mist spray

CAUTION: Cumin oil can irritate the skin and should either be avoided or used with extra care by people who have sensitive skin. Use small amounts. Cumin is photo-toxic. Avoid exposure to direct sunlight several hours after applying the oil on the skin.

CYPERUS (Cypriol)

Botanical Name: *Cyperus scariosus*
Family: *Cyperaceae*

The essential oil is obtained from the flowers and plant.

History and Information

- Cyperus is a sedge native to the Mediterranean region and Africa. The plant grows to a height of about 16 feet and has flowers. Cyperus is part of a species of six hundred plants growing in the tropics and subtropics.

- The plant was used by the Egyptians around 1550 B.C. to make a paper known as papyrus. The Egyptians also used the plant for making cloth and fragrancing.

Practical Uses

Warming; improves circulation
Calming, promotes a peaceful state of mind and restful sleep

Documented Properties

Decongestant, Hepatic, Insect Repellent, Tonic (*Digestive System*)

Aromatherapy Methods of Use: Application, aroma lamp, bath, inhaler, light bulb ring, massage, mist spray

CYPRESS

Botanical Name: *Cupressus sempervirens*
Family: *Cupressaceae*

The essential oil is obtained from the leaves and twigs of the tree.

History and Information

- Cypress is an evergreen tree native to Asia and the Mediterranean area. The tree grows to a height of about 160 feet. Some cypress trees are believed to be older than 3000 years.

- Early physicians recommended that patients with lung ailments go to the island of Crete, which had dense forests of cypress trees.

- The cypress plant contains a hormone that normalizes the female sex hormones and can be helpful during menopause.

Practical Uses

Purifying; helps in the reduction of cellulite
Balancing to the nervous system; calming, refreshing, relieves nervous tension and stress; promotes a restful sleep
Helps the breathing
Mood uplifting; improves mental clarity and alertness
Contracts weak connective tissue, relieves muscle tension
Lessens perspiration
Regulates the female reproductive and hormonal systems

Documented Properties

Antirheumatic, Antiseptic, Antispasmodic, Antisudorific, Antitussive, Astringent, Calmative, Cicatrizant, Deodorant, Deodorizer, Diuretic, Febrifuge, Hemostatic, Hepatic, Insect Repellent, Insecticide, Refreshing, Restorative (*Nervous System*), Sedative, Tonic, Vasoconstrictor, Warming

Aromatherapy Methods of Use: Application, aroma lamp, bath, diffusor, inhaler, light bulb ring, massage, mist spray, steam inhalation, steam and sauna room

DILL SEED & DILL WEED

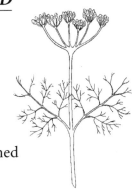

Botanical Name: *Anethum graveolens, Fructus anethi, Peucedanum graveolens*
Family: *Apiaceae*

Dill seed essential oil is obtained from the seeds. Dill weed essential oil is obtained from the whole plant.

History and Information

- Dill is native to the Mediterranean countries and Russia. The plant grows to a height of about 3 feet and has small yellow flowers.

- Writings found in Egyptian tombs show evidence that dill was used to help digestion.

- The Greek physician, Dioscorides, prescribed dill so frequently that it became known as the "herb of Dioscorides." Some of his recommended uses were for hiccoughs, flatulence, to increase lactation in nursing mothers, and stimulate urination.

- In medieval times, wounded knights placed dill seeds on their open cuts to speed the healing.

- Emperor Charlemagne insisted on having dill at his banquets as a remedy for hiccoughs and flatulence from indigestion.

- India's Ayurvedic and Unani practitioners use dill for indigestion, fever, and ulcers.

- Dill has been used over the centuries as an ingredient in exotic love potions and aphrodisiacs.

- The leaves and seeds have been used to increase lactation when taken daily by nursing mothers. Before they started nursing, mothers also rubbed their chest with dill seeds that were soaked in water.

- Since early times, dill has had a reputation of helping crying babies fall asleep.

- Dill has been used to sweeten bad breath.

- The seeds yield 2–4% essential oil.

Practical Uses

Improves digestion; soothes and freshens the intestines, relieves flatulence and fermentation
Calming, relaxing; promotes a restful sleep
Relieves pain and menstrual discomfort
Repels insects

Documented Properties

Antibacterial, Antispasmodic, Aperitive, Calmative, Carminative (*Prevents Flatulence and Fermentation and Stops Hiccoughs*), Detersive, Diaphoretic, Digestive, Disinfectant, Diuretic, Emmenagogue, Galactagogue, Laxative, Parasiticide, Resolvent, Sedative, Seductive, Stomachic

Aromatherapy Methods of Use: Application, aroma lamp, bath, diffusor, inhaler, light bulb ring, massage, mist spray

ELECAMPANE

Botanical Name: *Aster officinalis, Helenium grandiflorum, Inula helenium*
Family: *Asteraceae*

The essential oil is obtained from the root of the plant.

History and Information

- Elecampane is native to Europe and Asia. The plant grows to a height of about 4–8 feet and has large yellow, daisy-like flowers.

- Throughout history, the roots were eaten to relieve indigestion, asthma, and coughs.

- The ancient Greeks and Romans used elecampane as a remedy for colds, an expectorant, and to promote sweating. The Romans also ate the plant as a vegetable.

- The American Indians used the plant for bronchial and other lung ailments.

- In the 19th century, the roots were boiled in sugar water to make asthma lozenges, cough drops, and candy.

Practical Uses

Helps breathing
Mood uplifting

Documented Properties

Analgesic, Anthelmintic, Antibacterial, Antifungal, Anti-inflammatory, Antiseptic, Antispasmodic, Antitussive, Astringent, Carminative, Cholagogue, Diaphoretic, Digestive, Diuretic, Emmenagogue, Expectorant, Relaxant, Stimulant, Stomachic, Sudorific, Tonic, Vermifuge, Warming

Aromatherapy Methods of Use: Application, aroma lamp, inhaler, light bulb ring, massage, mist spray, steam inhalation, steam and sauna room

CAUTION: Elecampane oil can irritate the skin and should either be avoided or used with extra care by people who have sensitive skin. Use small amounts.

ELEMI

Botanical Name: *Canarium commune, C. luzonicum*
Family: *Burseraceae*

The resin/essential oil is obtained from the wood of the tree.

History and Information

- Elemi is an evergreen tree native to Asia. The tree grows to a height of about 80–100 feet and has yellow fragrant flowers that develop into green fruits with nuts called pili or philippine nut. These nuts are an important food source to millions of people. The tropical tree thrives in low elevations and warm climate and can bear up to 70 pounds of nuts annually. There are about seventy-five different varieties of pili nuts.

- The ancient Egyptians used elemi resin in the embalming process.

- In Europe during the 18th and 19th centuries, the aromatic resin of elemi was applied as an ointment to speed the healing of wounds.

- In Asia, the tree bark is used to treat malaria, while the lemon-scented resin is burned as an incense.

- The unroasted nuts are said to act as a purgative, while the roasted nuts are easily digestible. Infants are fed an emulsion of the powdered roasted nuts mixed with water as a substitute for milk.

- Pili nut oil is extracted from the nuts and has a high oil content of about 72%. These nuts do not store well and go rancid quickly.

- Elemi resin/oil is used as a perfume fixative to fragrance soaps, detergents, and cosmetics and to flavor foods and beverages.

Practical Uses

Warming; improves circulation
Calming, relaxing, reduces stress; promotes a restful sleep
Opens the breathing passages for deeper breathing, breaks up mucous (*mild effect*)
Mood uplifting; helps one to communicate inner feelings; helpful for meditation
Heals skin tissue

Documented Properties

Analgesic, Antibacterial, Antifungal, Antiseptic, Antiviral, Balsamic, Cicatrizant, Expectorant, Nervine, Stimulant (*Immune System*), Stomachic, Tonic, Vulnerary

Aromatherapy Methods of Use: Application, aroma lamp, bath, inhaler, light bulb ring, massage, mist spray, steam inhalation, steam and sauna room

EUCALYPTUS & EUCALYPTUS RADIATA

Botanical Name: *Eucalyptus globulus* (Eucalyptus); *Eucalyptus radiata* (Eucalyptus radiata)
Family: *Myrtaceae*

The essential oil is obtained from the leaves and twigs of the tree.

History and Information

- Eucalyptus globulus and eucalyptus radiata are native to Australia. Eucalyptus radiata grows to a height of about 170 feet. The eucalyptus globulus tree is one of the tallest trees—reaching over 300 feet to as high as 480 feet. The leaves are fragrant and leathery, the flowers are white, and the fruit is contained in a capsule. There are approximately seven hundred different species of eucalyptus. The tree is also known as the gum tree and its roots are said to store a large quantity of water in order to survive the dry seasons. The roots release a poisonous chemical that kills nearby plants.

- Eucalyptus has a long tradition of uses in medicine and is known to be an excellent antiseptic for purifying the environment. It became known as Catheter oil when British hospitals, in the 19th century, used it to sterilize urinary catheters.

- Historically, to improve their health, people who were sick were relocated to areas where the trees grew. In the latter part of the 19th century, eucalyptus oil was regarded as a cure-all.

- Koala bears feed exclusively on the leaves of the tree.

- The leaves yield approximately 2% essential oil.

Practical Uses

Cooling
Stimulating to the nervous system
Vapors open sinus and breathing passages, improves circulation
Refreshing, reviving, energizing; improves mental clarity and alertness
Relieves pain, aching and sore muscles
Disinfectant
Repels insects

Documented Properties

Analgesic, Anthelmintic, Antibacterial, Antidiabetic, Antidote, Antifungal, Anti-inflammatory, Antineuralgic, Antipruritic, Antiputrid, Antirheumatic, Antiseptic (*Strong*), Antispasmodic, Antivenomous, Antiviral (*Respiratory Tract*), Astringent, Balsamic, Cephalic, Cicatrizant, Cooling, Decon-

gestant, Deodorant, Deodorizer, Depurative, Diaphoretic, Disinfectant, Diuretic, Expectorant, Febrifuge, Germicide, Hemostatic, Insect Repellent, Insecticide, Invigorating, Parasiticide, Pectoral, Purifying, Regenerator (*Skin Tissue*), Rubefacient, Stimulant (*Circulatory System*), Tonic, Uplifting, Vermifuge, Vulnerary

Aromatherapy Methods of Use: Application, aroma lamp, bath, diffusor, inhaler, light bulb ring, massage, mist spray, steam inhalation, steam and sauna room

CAUTION: Due to the toxicity of eucalyptus oil, use small amounts. Eucalyptus radiata is considered to be non-toxic and safer to use than eucalyptus globulus.

EUCALYPTUS CITRIODORA

Botanical Name: *Eucalyptus citriodora*
Family: *Myrtaceae*

The essential oil is obtained from the leaves and twigs of the tree.

History and Information

- Eucalyptus citriodora is an evergreen tree native to Australia. The tree grows to a height of about 170 feet and has narrow pointed leaves. Every part of the tree has a strong lemony scent.

Practical Uses

Calming
Mood uplifting, reviving, helps to relieve a fatigued state

Documented Properties

Antibacterial, Antidepressant, Antifungal, Anti-inflammatory, Antirheumatic, Antiseptic, Antiviral, Calmative, Expectorant, Febrifuge, Insect Repellent, Pectoral, Sedative, Tonic, Vulnerary

Aromatherapy Methods of Use: Application, aroma lamp, diffusor, inhaler, light bulb ring, massage, mist spray

FENNEL

Botanical Name: *Anethum foeniculum, Foeniculum officinale, F. vulgare*
Family: *Apiaceae*

The essential oil is obtained from the seeds of the plant.

History and Information

- Fennel is native to Europe and Asia. The plant grows to a height of about 3–7 feet, and has dark green feathery leaves and clusters of small yellow flowers.

- The Romans and Greeks used the herb to lose weight. The Greeks also consumed fennel for courage and to prolong life. The Greek physicians, Hippocrates and Dioscorides, recommended fennel for nursing mothers to increase their lactation. Dioscorides also used fennel to suppress hunger, decrease fluid retention, and relieve inflammations related to the urinary system.

- Pliny, the Roman herbalist, recommended eating fennel to strengthen the eyesight. In later years, other herbalists corroborated with Pliny's findings, and prescribed extracts of the root to treat cataracts and the whole plant as a remedy for poor vision.

- The Hindus and Chinese used fennel as an antivenomous agent against snake and scorpion bites.

- Emperor Charlemagne ordered the herb grown in all of his imperial gardens.

- The household of King Edward I of England consumed more than 8 pounds of fennel a month.

- In China, the seeds are powdered and used as a poultice for snakebites.

- Fennel is said to stimulate the estrogen level, which is useful in helping women with sexual problems. It is also helpful for women who experience menstrual problems and premenstrual tension.

- Farmers have reported that adding fennel to the feed of nursing animals increases their lactation.

- The seeds yield 4–5% essential oil. Fennel oil is used as an ingredient in sour pickles, perfumes, soaps, cough syrups, licorice candy, and liqueurs. It has also been used as an ingredient in antiwrinkle creams for the skin.

Practical Uses

Warming; improves circulation
Improves digestion; soothes and purifies the intestines, relieves flatulence and aerophagy
Purifying; helps in the reduction of cellulite
Reduces stress; promotes a restful sleep
Helps the breathing
Relieves pain and menstrual discomfort
Increases lactation
Disinfectant
Repels insects

Documented Properties

Antibacterial, Antidote, Antiemetic, Antifungal, Antiphlogistic, Antiseptic, Antispasmodic, Antitoxic, Aperitif, Appetite Depressant, Astringent, Calmative, Carminative, Decongestant, Depurative, Detoxifier, Diaphoretic, Digestive, Diuretic, Emmenagogue, Estrogenic, Expectorant, Galactagogue, Hepatic, Insect Repellent, Insecticide, Laxative, Parasiticide, Regulator (*Female Reproductive System*), Resolvent, Revitalizing, Stimulant (*Uterine Contractions, Estrogen Levels*), Stomachic, Tonic, Vermifuge

Aromatherapy Methods of Use: Application, aroma lamp, bath, diffusor, inhaler, light bulb ring, massage, mist spray, steam inhalation, steam and sauna room

CAUTION: Due to the toxicity of the oil, use small amounts. Fennel oil can irritate the skin and should either be avoided or used with extra care by people who have sensitive skin. Fennel should not be used by people prone to epileptic seizures and people with kidney problems.

FIR BALSAM NEEDLES & FIR NEEDLES

Botanical Name: *Abies alba* (Silver fir*)*, *Abies balsamea* (Fir balsam needles), *Abies grandis* (Grand fir*)*, *Pseudotsuga menziesii* (Douglas fir)
Family: *Pinaceae*

The essential oil is obtained from the needles of the tree.

History and Information

- Fir is an evergreen tree native to North America and Europe. The trees range in height from 40–80 feet for the fir balsam and 100–300 feet for the fir needle. The leaves are needle-like, and the wood is soft and odorless. Fir trees are popularly used as a Christmas tree because their needles remain on the branches long after the tree has been cut. There are approximately forty species of the fir tree. The life span of the needles is up to 10 years.

- The American Indians used every part of the tree for a different remedy. The inner bark was prepared into a tea to alleviate chest pains; the twigs were used as a laxative; the roots were placed in the mouth to soothe sores; and the needles were used in sweat baths. Balsam needles and resin were placed in the sauna to help relieve colds and coughs. The resin was also applied on the skin to heal burns, sores, cuts, wounds, inflammation, congestion, and itching.

- The resin has been used as a source of turpentine, an adhesive for microscope slides and optical lenses, and an ingredient in hemorrhoid ointments. Dentists use the balsam to seal up root canals.

Practical Uses

Purifying; removes lymphatic deposits from the body; helps in the reduction of cellulite
Calming
Vapors open sinus and breathing passages
Mood uplifting, refreshing, reviving; improves mental clarity; encourages communication
Lessens pain

Documented Properties

Analgesic, Antiseptic, Antitussive, Astringent, Cicatrizant, Diuretic, Expectorant, Purgative, Sedative, Stimulant (*Respiratory System*), Tonic, Vulnerary

Aromatherapy Methods of Use: Application, aroma lamp, bath, inhaler, light bulb ring, massage, mist spray, steam inhalation, steam and sauna room

FIR BALSAM RESIN

Botanical Name: *Abies balsamea, A. balsamifera, Pinus balsaamea*
Family: *Pinaceae*

The resin is obtained from the inner bark of the tree.

History and Information

See fir balsam needles.

Practical Uses

Warming; improves circulation
Purifying; helps in the reduction of cellulite
Calming; promotes a restful sleep
Mood uplifting
Reduces and soothes swollen tissue
Soothes insect bites

Documented Properties

Antiscorbutic, Antiseptic, Expectorant, Pectoral, Sedative, Tonic, Vulnerary, Warming

Aromatherapy Methods of Use: Application, massage

FRANKINCENSE (Olibanum)

Botanical Name: *Boswellia carteri*, *B. thurifera*
Family: *Burseraceae*

The resin/essential oil is obtained from the bark of the tree.

History and Information

- Frankincense is native to the Mediterranean area. The small tree grows to a height of about 20 feet and has white flowers.

- Nearly 5000 years ago, the ancient Egyptians burned the incense of frankincense in the temples during religious ceremonies and later used the gum as a facial mask to rejuvenate their skin.

- Traditionally, frankincense was used to fumigate sickrooms. The Chinese used the gum in the treatment of leprosy and tuberculosis.

- The yield of essential oil is approximately 5%. The oil is used as an ingredient in Oriental perfumes, soaps, and cosmetics. The incense is still burned in many of today's churches.

Practical Uses

Calming, relaxing; promotes a restful sleep
Vapors open sinus and breathing passages
Mood uplifting, brings out feelings; helpful for meditation
Reduces inflammation
Soothes and heals inflamed skin; bruises, burns

Documented Properties

Analgesic, Antibacterial, Antidepressant, Anti-inflammatory, Antiseptic, Antispasmodic, Antitussive, Astringent, Balsamic, Carminative, Cephalic, Cicatrizant, Cytophylactic, Digestive, Diuretic, Emollient, Emmenagogue, Expectorant, Fixative, Nervine, Pectoral, Rejuvenator (*Skin*), Revitalizing, Sedative, Stimulant (*Cells, Immune System*), Tonic, Tonifying (*Skin*), Uplifting, Vulnerary, Warming

Aromatherapy Methods of Use: Application, aroma lamp, bath, diffusor, inhaler, light bulb ring, massage, mist spray, steam inhalation, steam and sauna room

GALANGAL

Botanical Name: *Alpinia officinarum, Languas officinarum*
Family: *Zingiberaceae*

The essential oil is obtained from the plant roots.

History and Information

- Galangal is native to China. The plant grows to a height of about 5 feet, and has green sword-

shaped leaves, white flowers, and an aromatic rhizome.

- During the Middle Ages, galangal was used as an aphrodisiac.

- In Asian cooking, the rhizome is substituted for ginger while the shoots and flowers are eaten fresh in a salad or cooked. Galangal is also used as a remedy for cholera, congestion, digestion, and skin problems.

Practical Uses

Improves digestion
Reduces stress
Mood uplifting
Relieves aches and pains
General stimulant
Disinfectant

Documented Properties

Analgesic, Anti-inflammatory, Antiseptic, Anti-spasmodic, Antitussive, Aphrodisiac, Balsamic, Carminative, Cicatrizant, Digestive, Diuretic, Emmenagogue, Expectorant, Hypotensive, Restorative, Stimulant, Stomachic, Tonic

Aromatherapy Methods of Use: Application, aroma lamp, diffusor, inhaler, light bulb ring, massage, mist spray

COMMENTS: Galangal oil is relatively expensive and can be substituted with ginger oil.

GALBANUM

Botanical Name: *Ferula galbaniflua, F. gummosa, F. rubicaulis*
Family: *Apiaceae*

The resin/essential oil is obtained from the bark of the plant.

History and Information

- Galbanum is native to the Mediterranean region. The thin and resinous plant grows to a height of about 3 feet, and has long grayish-green hairy leaves and umbels of very small yellow flowers that bear seeds.

- Galbanum is mentioned in the Bible as one of the ingredients in the holy ointment. It was also used by the Greeks, Hippocrates, and Pliny, the Roman herbalist.

Practical Uses

Calming; reduces stress
Mood uplifting
Relieves pain and inflammation

Documented Properties

Analgesic, Anti-inflammatory, Antiseptic, Antispasmodic, Aphrodisiac, Balsamic, Carminative, Cicatrizant, Digestive, Diuretic, Emmenagogue, Expectorant, Hypotensive, Nervine, Resolvent, Restorative, Stimulant, Tonic, Vulnerary

Aromatherapy Methods of Use: Application, aroma lamp, bath, inhaler, light bulb ring, massage, mist spray

GARDENIA

Botanical Name: *Gardenia grandiflora*
Family: *Rubiaceae*

The absolute/essential oil is obtained from the flowers of the bush.

History and Information

- Gardenia is an evergreen bush native to Asia. The plant grows to a height of about 10 feet and has fragrant waxy-white flowers that develop into orange fruits.

- In China, the flowers are used to scent tea; the roots and leaves are used to reduce fevers and cleanse the body.

- In Africa, the fruits are used as a spice in cooking.

- In Thailand, a yellow food-coloring is made from the fruits.

Practical Uses

Mood uplifting

Documented Properties

Alterative, Analgesic, Anthelmintic, Antibacterial, Anticonvulsive, Antidepressant, Anti-inflammatory, Antiseptic, Aphrodisiac, Calmative, Choleretic, Febrifuge, Hemostatic, Hepatic, Hypnotic, Hypotensor, Sedative, Stomachic, Uplifting

Aromatherapy Methods of Use: Application, aroma lamp, bath, fragrancing, light bulb ring, massage, mist spray

GERANIUM

Botanical Name: *Pelargonium graveolens*
Family: *Geraniaceae*

The essential oil is obtained from the leaves, stems, and flowers of the plant.

History and Information

- Geranium is a small fragrant plant native to Africa. The plant grows to a height of about 3 feet. There are over seven hundred different species of geranium.

- In ancient times, geranium was regarded as an exceptional healing agent for wounds and fractures.

- The American Indians drank a tea made from the powdered roots for dysentery, hemorrhaging, and ulcers. Poultices were made from the same preparation for hemorrhoids and arthritis.

- Early American women regularly drank a tea made from the roots, which was thought to prevent pregnancy.

Practical Uses

Cooling
Purifying; helps in the reduction of cellulite
Calming to the nervous system in small amounts and stimulating in large amounts; reduces tension
Mood uplifting; encourages communication
Lessens pain and inflammation
Stimulates the adrenal glands
Disinfectant
Repels insects
Soothes insect bites, lice, ticks

Documented Properties

Analgesic, Antibacterial, Anticoagulant, Antidepressant, Antidiabetic, Antifungal, Anti-inflammatory, Antineuralgic, Antiseptic, Antispasmodic, Antistress, Astringent, Cicatrizant, Cytophylactic, Deodorant, Depurative, Diuretic, Healing, Hemostatic, Insect Repellent, Insecticide, Parasiticide, Protectant (*Cells*), Refreshing, Rejuvenator (*Skin Tissue*), Regulator (*Glandular Functions and Hormones*), Sedative (*Mild*) (*Anxiety*), Stimulant (*Adrenal Glands; Circulatory and Lymphatic Systems*), Tonic, Tonifying (*Skin*), Uplifting (*Menopause and Premenstrual Tension*), Vasoconstrictor, Vermifuge, Vulnerary

Aromatherapy Methods of Use: Application, aroma lamp, bath, diffusor, inhaler, light bulb ring, massage, mist spray

GINGER

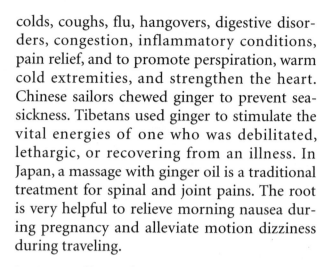

Botanical Name: *Zingiber officinale*
Family: *Zingiberaceae*

The essential oil is obtained from the roots of the plant.

History and Information

- Ginger is native to Asia. The plant grows to a height of about 3 feet, and has white or yellow flowers.

- The ancient people of India used ginger in cooking, to preserve food, and treat digestive problems.

- Dioscorides, the Greek physician, recommended the root to aid digestion and as a poison antidote. The Romans and Greeks later also used ginger to improve digestion.

- In the 16th century, Henry VIII recommended ginger root as a remedy for the plague.

- In Oriental medicine, ginger root is incorporated in about half of the herbal formulations. In China, the herb has been used for thousands of years as a general tonic, a remedy for colds, coughs, flu, hangovers, digestive disorders, congestion, inflammatory conditions, pain relief, and to promote perspiration, warm cold extremities, and strengthen the heart. Chinese sailors chewed ginger to prevent seasickness. Tibetans used ginger to stimulate the vital energies of one who was debilitated, lethargic, or recovering from an illness. In Japan, a massage with ginger oil is a traditional treatment for spinal and joint pains. The root is very helpful to relieve morning nausea during pregnancy and alleviate motion dizziness during traveling.

- In Ayurvedic medicine, ginger was employed as a remedy for liver problems, intestinal gas, hemorrhoids, and anemia.

- Herbalists have recommended compresses of hot ginger to relieve gout, headaches, aches and pains, sinus congestion, and menstrual cramps. A warm ginger footbath is said to invigorate the entire body.

- East Africans use ginger for headaches and parasites. It is said to be effective against intestinal roundworms.

- The root yields 1–3% essential oil. Ginger is an ingredient in perfumery as well as an additive in foods, ginger ale, and ginger beer. It is significantly used as an antioxidant in food products.

Practical Uses

Warming; improves circulation
Improves digestion; soothes the intestines, relieves flatulence
Mood uplifting, improves mental clarity and memory
General stimulant to the entire body; relieves dizziness and nausea caused by traveling
Relieves aches and pains
Cleanses the bowels
Disinfectant

Documented Properties

Analgesic, Antibacterial, Anticoagulant, Antiemetic, Antioxidant, Antiscorbutic, Antiseptic, Antispasmodic, Antitussive, Antitoxic, Aperitif, Aperitive, Aphrodisiac, Astringent (*Stops Bleeding*), Carminative, Cephalic, Diaphoretic, Digestive (*Nausea*), Diuretic, Emmenagogue, Expectorant, Febrifuge, Laxative, Rubefacient, Stimulant (*Circulatory and Nervous Systems*), Stomachic, Tonic, Tonifying (*Digestive System*), Vermifuge

Aromatherapy Methods of Use: Application, aroma lamp, diffusor, inhaler, light bulb ring, massage, mist spray

CAUTION: Ginger oil can irritate the skin and should either be avoided or used with extra care by people who have sensitive skin. Use small amounts.

GINGERGRASS

Botanical Name: *Cymbopogon martinii* var. *sofia*
Family: *Poaceae*

The essential oil is obtained from the plant, which is a grass.

History and Information

- Gingergrass is a grass native to Asia and thrives in moist soils. The plant is closely related to palmarosa.

Practical Uses

Warming; improves circulation
Calming; reduces stress
Vapors open sinus and breathing passages
Mood uplifting, aphrodisiac, euphoric; improves mental clarity

Documented Properties

Antibacterial, Antifungal, Antiviral, Tonic

Aromatherapy Methods of Use: Application, aroma lamp, diffusor, inhaler, light bulb ring, massage, mist spray

CAUTION: Gingergrass oil can irritate the skin and should either be avoided or used with extra care by people who have sensitive skin. Use small amounts.

GOLDENROD

Botanical Name: *Solidago canadensis, S. odora*
Family: *Asteraceae*

The essential oil is obtained from the flower of the plant.

History and Information

- Goldenrod is native to North America. The plant grows to a height of 3–7 feet, and has thin leaves and yellow flowers.

- The American Indians made a lotion from the flowers for bee stings. The roots were taken for liver problems.

- Early American settlers used the flowers to help the gums and teeth.

- In Europe, the flowers are taken as a laxative, and for sinus and joint problems. The seeds are used for diarrhea.

- The herb was made as a tea during the American revolt against the British tea tax. The tea was known as "patriot tea."

- In Chinese medicine, the herb is used for malaria, headaches, and sore throats.

- Herbalists use goldenrod leaves for wounds, abrasions, and insect bites.

Practical Uses

Warming; improves circulation
Calming; reduces stress
Mood uplifting, improves mental clarity, encourages communication, helpful for meditation
Relieves pain

Documented Properties

Analgesic, Astringent, Carminative, Diaphoretic, Diuretic, Hepatic, Laxative, Tonic

Aromatherapy Methods of Use: Application, aroma lamp, bath, diffusor, light bulb ring, inhaler, massage, mist spray

GRAPEFRUIT

Botanical Name: *Citrus paradisi, C. racemosa*
Family: *Rutaceae*

The essential oil is obtained from the peel of the fruit.

History and Information

- Grapefruit is an evergreen citrus tree that grows to a height of about 30–50 feet and has fragrant white flowers. The earliest record of the grapefruit is in the West Indies in the early 18th century. Scientists believe that the tree developed as a mutation from the pomelo fruit. The first grapefruit trees in Florida were planted in about 1820.

- The peel contains a bitter component called naringin, which is used as a flavoring in chocolate and bitter tonic beverages. The seeds produce grapefruit seed oil, which is a dark, bitter oil. When refined to extract the bitter taste, the seed oil can be used in salads and as a cooking oil.

Practical Uses

Cooling
Purifying; reduces cellulite and obesity; balances the fluids in the body
Reduces stress
Mood uplifting, refreshing, reviving; improves mental clarity and awareness, sharpens the senses
Increases physical strength and energy

Documented Properties

Antibacterial, Antidepressant, Antiseptic, Anti-stress, Antitoxic, Aperitif, Aperitive, Astringent, Balancing (*Central Nervous System*), Cephalic, Cholagogue, Depurative, Detoxifier, Digestive, Disinfectant, Diuretic, Hemostatic, Resolvent, Restorative, Reviving, Stimulant (*Digestive and Lymphatic Systems, and Neurotransmitters*), Tonic (*Liver*), Tonifying (*Skin*)

Aromatherapy Methods of Use: Application, aroma lamp, bath, diffusor, inhaler, light bulb ring, massage, mist spray

CAUTION: Grapefruit oil can irritate the skin and should either be avoided or used with extra care by people who have sensitive skin. Use small amounts. Grapefruit is phototoxic. Avoid exposure to direct sunlight several hours after applying the oil on the skin.

GUAIACWOOD

Botanical Name: *Bulnesia sarmienti, Guaiacum officinale*
Family: *Zygophyllaceae*

The resin/essential oil is obtained from the wood of the tree.

History and Information

- Guaiacwood is an evergreen tree native to the West Indies and Central America. The tree grows to a height of about 40 feet, and has leathery leaves and blue or purple flowers. Guaiacwood is also known as guaiacum, guay-acan, pockwood, and Lignum vitae, which means "wood of life." The wood of the tree has a rich supply of fats and resins that make it very hard and impervious to water.

- During the 16th century, guaiacwood was widely used for the treatment of syphilis.

Practical Uses

Purifying to the tissues
Calming and relaxing; reduces stress and tension, promotes a restful sleep
Mood uplifting; improves mental clarity; helpful for meditation
Reduces inflammation; loosens tight muscles
Soothes swollen and injured skin tissue

Documented Properties

Anti-inflammatory, Antirheumatic, Antiseptic, Aphrodisiac, Astringent, Balsamic, Diaphoretic, Diuretic, Laxative, Stimulant (*Genitourinary System*), Sudorific, Tonifying (*Skin*)

Aromatherapy Methods of Use: Application, aroma lamp, bath, light bulb ring, massage, mist spray

HELICHRYSUM (*Everlasting or Immortelle*)

Botanical Name: *Helichrysum angustifolium, H. italicum*
Family: *Asteraceae*

The essential oil is obtained from the flowers of the plant.

History and Information

- Helichrysum is an evergreen plant native to the Mediterranean area and Asia. The plant grows to a height of about 2 feet and has daisy-like yellow flowers. There are approximately five hundred species of helichrysum.

- The plant was used in Europe over the years to freshen the air, repel insects, and for medicinal purposes.

Practical Uses

Cooling
Relaxing; reduces stress
Vapors open the sinus and breathing passages
Mood uplifting, euphoric, reviving, strengthening, improves mental clarity and alertness
Relieves aches, pains and menstrual discomfort
Increases muscle endurance
Disinfectant

Documented Properties

Analgesic, Antibacterial, Anticoagulant, Antidepressant, Antifungal, Anti-inflammatory, Antiseptic, Antispasmodic, Antistress, Antitussive, Antiviral, Astringent, Blood Purifier, Cephalic, Cicatrizant, Cholagogue, Cytophylactic, Detoxifier, Diuretic, Emollient, Expectorant, Hepatic, Nervine, Regenerator (*Skin Cells*), Sedative, Stimulant (*Dreaming*), Tonic

Aromatherapy Methods of Use: Application, aroma lamp, bath, light bulb ring, inhaler, massage, mist spray, steam inhalation, steam and sauna room

HOPS

Botanical Name: *Humulus lupulus*
Family: *Moraceae*

The essential oil is obtained from the buds and flowers of the plant.

History and Information

- Hops is a climbing vine native to Europe and Asia. The plant grows to about 19–25 feet and has pale green, bell-shaped flowers. The male and female flowers grow on separate plants. Hops belongs to the same family as marijuana.

- The Romans ate the shoots of the plant as a vegetable.

- During the 9th and 10th centuries, brewers in Germany and France widely used hops as a preservative in the beer they produced.

- Herbalists mixed hops into their herbal remedies to stimulate estrogen production, relieve pain, and in the treatment of insomnia, rheumatism, jaundice, and other conditions.

- The female flowers contain cone-like catkins that ripen into small egg-shaped fruiting cones. Brewers use the whole cones to give beer a bitter taste and calming effect.

Practical Uses

Calming; promotes a restful sleep
Mild pain reliever

Documented Properties

Analgesic, Antibacterial, Anticonvulsive, Anti-inflammatory, Antilithic, Antipruritic, Antispasmodic, Aperitive, Aphrodisiac (*For Women*), Astringent, Blood Purifier, Calmative, Carminative, Digestive, Diuretic, Emmenagogue, Emollient, Estrogenic, Febrifuge, Galactagogue, Hepatic, Hypnotic, Nervine, Sedative, Sudorific, Tonic, Tranquilizer, Vermifuge

Aromatherapy Methods of Use: Application, massage, mist spray

COMMENTS: The fresh hops fruits can cause hypersomnia, vomiting, profuse perspiration, overexcitement, and dermatitis.

CAUTION: Hops oil is moderately toxic. Use small amounts.

HYSSOP

Botanical Name: *Hyssopus officinalis* (Hyssop); *Hyssop officinalis* var. *decumbens* (Hyssop decumbens)
Family: *Lamiaceae*

The essential oil is obtained from the leaves and flowering tops of the plant.

History and Information

- Hyssop is a semi-evergreen plant native to Europe and Asia. The bushy plant grows to a height of about 1–4 feet, and has aromatic leaves and spikes of white, pink, blue, or dark purple flowers.

- In ancient times, the herb was used to fragrantly scent and purify the air during religious services and celebrations. An ancient pharmacopoeia mentioned hyssop as the major ingredient in numerous preparations, elixirs, and syrups.

- Hyssop was prescribed by Hippocrates, Galen, and Dioscorides for its healing effects on the respiratory system.

- In the 16th and 17th centuries, herbalists used the plant to soothe coughs and congestion.

- In England, hyssop baths were taken to relieve aching muscles and joints.

- The strong fragrance of hyssop attracts bees and adds a sweet smell to the honey.

Practical Uses

Relaxing
Vapors open the sinus and breathing passages
Mood uplifting, reviving; improves mental clarity and alertness
Used in perfumery

Documented Properties

Antibacterial, Anti-inflammatory, Antirheumatic, Antiseptic, Antispasmodic, Antiviral, Aperient, Astringent, Balsamic, Cardiac, Carminative, Cephalic, Cicatrizant, Depurative, Diaphoretic, Digestive, Diuretic, Emmenagogue, Emollient, Expectorant, Febrifuge, Healing (*Skin*), Hypertensor, Laxative (*Mild*), Nervine, Parasiticide, Pectoral, Regulator (*Blood Pressure*), Resolvent, Stimulant (*Adrenal Glands*), Stomachic, Sudorific, Tonic, Vermifuge, Vulnerary

Aromatherapy Methods of Use: Application, aroma lamp, diffusor, inhaler, light bulb ring, massage, mist spray, steam inhalation, steam and sauna room

CAUTION: Due to the toxicity of the oil, use small amounts. Hyssop should not be used by people who are prone to epileptic seizures. The oil from the variety of *Hyssop decumbens* is less toxic than other hyssop oils.

JASMINE

Botanical Name:
Jasminum officinale
Family: *Oleaceae*

The absolute/essential oil is obtained from the flower petals of the bush.

History and Information

- Jasmine is native to Asia and belongs to the olive family. The bush grows to a height of about 40 feet and has fragrant white flowers.

- Persian women soaked jasmine flowers in sesame oil to massage into their body and hair.

- The Chinese so highly prize the fragrance of jasmine that they use the flowers to scent beverages, cosmetics, massage oils, and to freshen the air. Medicinally, the flowers are used for liver problems and as a blood purifier. The root is used for insomnia, headaches, and other pains.

- Jasmine flowers are picked after the sun has set to capture their aromatic scent.

- Jasmine garlands are used in Buddhist ceremonies to symbolize respect.

Practical Uses

Mood uplifting, aphrodisiac

Documented Properties

Analgesic, Antidepressant, Anti-inflammatory, Antipruritic, Antiseptic, Antispasmodic, Anti-stress, Aphrodisiac, Calmative, Carminative, Cicatrizant, Decongestant, Emollient, Euphoriant, Expectorant, Galactagogue, Moisturizer (*Skin*), Rejuvenator (*Skin*), Sedative, Stimulant (*Uterine Contractions*), Tonic (*Female Reproductive System*), Uplifting

Aromatherapy Methods of Use: Application, aroma lamp, bath, fragrancing, light bulb ring, massage, mist spray

JUNIPER BERRIES

Botanical Name: *Juniperus communis*
Family: *Cupressaceae*

The essential oil is obtained from the ripe berries of the bush.

History and Information

- Juniper is an evergreen bush native to Europe, Asia and the northern hemisphere. The bush is about 2–6 feet in height and sometimes reaches as high as 25 feet. The male trees have yellow cones and the female trees have bluish-green cones. The silvery-green leaves are needle-like. The green berries take 3 years to ripen to a blue color. The maximum life span of the bush is 2000 years.

- The Romans used the berries as an antiseptic and to flavor foods.

- In the Middle Ages, juniper was burned to protect people against the plague.

- The tree was a source of food for the American Indians. They ate the inner bark, ground up the berries to make cakes, and made a tea from the leaves. The berries were combined with the twigs to make a tea high in vitamin C. For medicinal uses, a tea was brewed from the juniper twigs to cure stomachaches and colds; the berries were used as a blood tonic and applied topically to stop bleeding and heal wounds. During and after illnesses, the branches were burned to fumigate the living quarters. Inhalation of the smoke was also used to help respiratory problems. Every part of the tree was used as an antiseptic.

- In folk medicine the berries were infused in water and used as an antidote for poisonous bites. In Europe, juniper was regarded as helpful to expel worms, and for cholera and typhoid.

- The berries are used to make gin. They are also roasted and used as a coffee substitute.

Practical Uses

Purifying; helps in the reduction of cellulite; cleansing to the intestines and the tissues in the body
Relaxing, reduces stress
Mood uplifting, refreshing, reviving; improves mental clarity and memory
Lessens pain, painful swellings; painful menstruation, fluid retention
Disinfectant
Repels insects
Soothes insect bites

Documented Properties

Analgesic, Antifungal, Antilithic, Antirheumatic, Antiscorbutic, Antiseptic, Antispasmodic, Antitoxic, Aphrodisiac, Astringent, Blood Purifier, Carminative, Cicatrizant, Cholagogue, Depurative, Detoxifier, Disinfectant, Diuretic (*Strong*), Emmenagogue, Expectorant, Healing, Hemostatic, Insecticide, Nervine, Parasiticide, Refreshing, Rubefacient, Sedative, Stimulant (*Genitourinary Tract*), Stomachic, Sudorific, Tonic, Tonifying, Vermifuge, Vulnerary

Aromatherapy Methods of Use: Application, aroma lamp, bath, diffusor, inhaler, light bulb ring, massage, mist spray

CAUTION: Due to juniper's strong stimulating effect on the kidneys, use small amounts. Avoid use on a person who has weak kidneys.

LABDANUM (Cistus or Rock Rose)

Botanical Name: *Cistus ladanifer*
Family: *Cistaceae*

The resin/essential oil is obtained from the leaves of the bush.

History and Information

- Labdanum is a small evergreen bush native to the Mediterranean area and Middle East. The bush grows to a height of about 10 feet and has large white flowers.

- Labdanum is used in expensive perfumes because of its excellent fixative qualities.

Practical Uses

Warming; increases circulation
Calming; reduces stress, promotes a restful sleep
Mood uplifting, euphoric; brings out feelings, encourages communication; helpful for meditation
Loosens tight muscles
Used as a fixative to hold the scent of a fragrance

Documented Properties

Antiarthritic, Anticoagulant, Antiseptic, Antispasmodic, Antitussive, Astringent, Balsamic, Cicatrizant, Depurative, Diuretic, Drying, Emmenagogue, Expectorant, Fixative, Insecticide, Sedative, Tonic, Vulnerary

Aromatherapy Methods of Use: Application, aroma lamp, inhaler, light bulb ring, massage, mist spray

LANTANA

Botanical Name: *Lantana camara*
Family: *Verbenaceae*

The essential oil is obtained from the leaves of the shrub.

History and Information

- Lantana is a vigorous-growing shrub native to the United States that reaches a height of about 6 feet. The flowers are orange and develop into black berries. The berries and dry leaves are poisonous.

Practical Uses

Cooling
Calming, reduces stress; promotes a restful sleep
Mood uplifting

Documented Properties

Antispasmodic, Antiviral, Cicatrizant, Emmenagogue, Febrifuge

Aromatherapy Methods of Use: Application, aroma lamp, bath, inhaler, light bulb ring, massage, mist spray

CAUTION: Lantana oil is moderately toxic. Use small amounts.

LARCH

Botanical Name: *Larix europaea*
Family: *Pinaceae*

The essential oil is obtained from the needles of the tree.

History and Information

- Larch is a deciduous conifer native to the northern hemisphere. The tree is one of the fastest growing of all trees and reaches a height of about 65 feet. It has soft needle-like leaves and bears a flower called the larch rose. The wood is strong and durable.

Practical Uses

Vapors open the sinus and breathing passages
Mood uplifting

Documented Properties

Analgesic, Antidepressant, Antiseptic, Astringent, Diuretic, Hemostatic, Laxative, Vulnerary

Aromatherapy Methods of Use: Aroma lamp, inhaler, light bulb ring, mist spray, steam inhalation, steam and sauna room

CAUTION: Larch oil is toxic. Use in small amounts.

LAVANDIN

Botanical Name: *Lavandula fragrans, L. hortensis, L. hybrida*
Family: *Lamiaceae*

The essential oil is obtained from the flowers of the plant.

History and Information

- Lavandin is an evergreen plant native to the Mediterranean area. The plant grows to a height of about 3 feet and has lilac-colored flowers.

- Lavandin is a hybrid plant of lavender. The hybridization occurs naturally by the work of bees. Compared to lavender, the lavandin plant has greater resistance to disease and can tolerate harsher weather conditions. It also produces a greater number of flowers and approximately four times the amount of oil, but of a lower grade. Lavandin oil is less expensive than lavender oil, but it is often sold falsely as lavender.

Practical Uses

Improves digestion; soothing to the intestines
Purifying; helps in the reduction of cellulite
Calming and strengthening to the nerves, relaxes the muscles, promotes a restful sleep
Calming in small amounts and stimulates the nervous system in large amounts
Vapors open sinus and breathing passages
Mood uplifting; balances mood swings
Lessens aches and pains; gently reduces fluid retention
Disinfectant
Repels insects, kills parasites and lice

Healing to the skin: Bruises, cuts, wounds, burns, sunburn, scars, sores, insect bites, and injuries

Documented Properties

Analgesic, Anticonvulsive, Antidepressant, Antirheumatic, Antiseptic, Antitoxic, Carminative, Cholagogue, Choleretic, Cicatrizant, Cordial, Cytophylactic, Deodorant, Deodorizer, Disinfectant, Diuretic, Emmenagogue, Expectorant, Hypotensor, Insect Repellent, Nervine, Parasiticide, Sedative, Stimulant (*Respiratory System*), Sudorific, Tonic, Vermifuge, Vulnerary

Aromatherapy Methods of Use: Application, aroma lamp, bath, diffusor, inhaler, light bulb ring, massage, mist spray, steam inhalation, steam and sauna room

LAVENDER

Botanical Name: *Lavandula augustifolia, L. officinalis, L. vera*
Family: *Lamiaceae*

The essential oil is obtained from the flowers of the plant.

History and Information

- Lavender is an evergreen plant native to the Mediterranean area. The plant grows to a height of about 3 feet and has lilac-colored flowers. There are twenty-eight species of this plant.

- Lavender is regarded as one of the most useful and versatile essences for therapeutic purposes. Herbalists have used the essential oil for head pains, loss of consciousness, and cramps. Lavender's relaxing properties are used on lions and tigers in zoos to keep them calm. Lavender is also known to have a powerful anti-venom property that starts neutralizing the poison of a snake or insect bite immediately after it is applied.

Practical Uses

Improves digestion; soothing to the intestines
Purifying; helps in the reduction of cellulite
Calming and strengthening to the nerves, relaxes the muscles, lessens tension, promotes a restful sleep
Calming in small amounts and stimulating to the nervous system in large amounts
Vapors open sinus and breathing passages
Mood uplifting; balances mood swings
Lessens aches and pains; gently removes fluid retention
Disinfectant
Repels insects, kills parasites and lice

Healing to the skin: Bruises, cuts, wounds, burns, sunburns, scars, sores, insect bites, and injuries

Documented Properties

Analgesic, Antibacterial, Anticonvulsive, Antidepressant (*Premenstrual Syndrome and Menopause*), Antifungal, Anti-inflammatory, Antirheumatic, Antiseptic, Antispasmodic, Antistress, Antitoxic, Antitussive, Antivenomous, Antiviral, Aperitive, Calmative, Carminative, Cephalic, Cholagogue, Cicatrizant, Cordial, Cytophylactic, Decongestant, Deodorant, Detoxifier, Diuretic, Emmenagogue, Healing (*Skin*), Hypotensor, Insect Repellent, Nervine, Parasiticide, Regenerator (*Skin Tissue*), Restorative, Reviving, Sedative (*Heart*), Stimulant (*Respiratory System*), Stomachic, Sudorific, Tonic, Vermifuge, Vulnerary

Aromatherapy Methods of Use: Application, aroma lamp, bath, diffusor, inhaler, light bulb ring, massage, mist spray, steam inhalation, steam and sauna room

LEDUM GROENLANDICUM

Botanical Name: *Ledum groenlandicum*
Family: *Ericaceae*

The essential oil is obtained from the leaves of the shrub.

History and Information

- Ledum Groenlandicum is an evergreen shrub native to North America. The shrub grows to a height of about 3 feet, and has leathery leaves and clusters of white fragrant flowers.

- The native Canadian people brewed a tea from the leaves called labrador tea. The tea was used as an expectorant and for colds.

Practical Uses

Warming; improves circulation
Calming; reduces stress
Improves mental clarity and alertness; helpful for meditation

Documented Properties

Analgesic, Antibacterial, Anti-inflammatory, Antiseptic, Antispasmodic, Decongestant, Diaphoretic, Digestive, Diuretic, Emmenagogue, Expectorant, Febrifuge, Hepatic, Insecticide, Stimulant, Stomachic

Aromatherapy Methods of Use: Application, aroma lamp, bath, diffusor, inhaler, light bulb ring, massage, mist spray

CAUTION: Due to the relaxing effect of the oil, ledum should not be used before driving or doing anything that requires full attention.

LEMON

Botanical Name: *Citrus limon*
Family: *Rutaceae*

The essential oil is obtained from the peel of the fruit of the tree.

History and Information

- Lemon is an evergreen citrus tree native to Asia. The tree grows to a height of about 10–20 feet and has fragrant white flowers.

- The Greeks used lemon to perfume clothing.

- In England, lemon oil is used in the hospitals to freshen the air and neutralize unpleasant body odors. It is also used to strengthen the emotional states of depressed and fearful patients.

Practical Uses

Cooling
Purifying; breaks down cellulite, cleanses the tissues
Calming, relaxing, reduces stress; promotes a restful sleep
Mood uplifting, refreshing, reviving; improves mental clarity, alertness, and memory; sharpens the senses
Disinfectant
Soothes insect bites

Documented Properties

Antianemic, Antibacterial, Antidepressant, Antifungal, Antilithic, Antineuralgic, Antipruritic, Antirheumatic, Antisclerotic, Antiscorbutic, Antiseptic (*Strong*), Antispasmodic, Antistress, Antitoxic, Antitussive, Aperitive, Astringent, Blood Purifier, Calmative, Carminative, Cephalic, Cicatrizant, Coagulant, Cooling, Decongestant, Depurative, Detoxifier, Diaphoretic, Digestive, Disinfectant, Diuretic, Emollient, Febrifuge, Hemostatic, Hepatic, Hypotensor, Insect Repellent, Insecticide, Invigorating (*Immune System*), Laxative, Parasiticide, Refreshing, Rubefacient, Sedative, Stimulant (*Circulatory and Lymphatic Systems*), Stomachic, Tonic, Uplifting, Vermifuge

Aromatherapy Methods of Use: Application, aroma lamp, bath, diffusor, inhaler, light bulb ring, massage, mist spray

CAUTION: Lemon oil can irritate the skin and should either be avoided or used with extra care by people who have sensitive skin. Use small amounts. Lemon is phototoxic. Avoid exposure to direct sunlight several hours after applying the oil on the skin.

LEMON VERBENA

Botanical Name: *Aloysia citriodora, A. triphylla, Lippia citriodora, L. triphylla, Verbena triphylla*
Family: *Verbenaceae*

The essential oil is obtained from the leaves and branches of the bush.

History and Information

- Lemon verbena is native to South America. The bush grows to a height of about 6–10 feet, and has strong lemon-scented leaves and small white or purple blossoms that have a tiny yellow dot in the center. When touched, the flower releases a refreshing fragrance.

- The oil is an ingredient in perfumes and liqueurs. Lemon verbena oil is rare and expensive, and frequently adulterated with cheaper oils like citronella or lemongrass.

Practical Uses

Mood uplifting, reviving; improves mental clarity and alertness

Documented Properties

Antidepressant, Antiseptic, Antispasmodic, Aphrodisiac, Aperitive, Calmative, Carminative, Cholagogue, Cooling, Detoxifier, Digestive, Diuretic, Emollient, Febrifuge, Galactagogue, Hepatic, Insect Repellent, Insecticide, Nervine, Refreshing, Sedative, Stimulant(*Circulatory System*), Stomachic, Tonic (*Nerves*), Tonifying (*Skin*), Uplifting

Aromatherapy Methods of Use: Application, aroma lamp, inhaler, light bulb ring, massage, mist spray

CAUTION: Lemon verbena oil can irritate the skin and should either be avoided or used with extra care by people who have sensitive skin. Use small amounts. Lemon verbena is phototoxic. Avoid exposure to direct sunlight several hours after applying the oil on the skin.

LEMONGRASS

Botanical Name: *Cymbopogon citratus, C. flexuosus*
Family: *Poaceae*

The essential oil is obtained from the whole plant.

History and Information

- Lemongrass is native to Asia. The grass grows to a height of about 2 feet, and has bulbous stems and sword-like leaves.

- In India, the oil is applied on the skin for ringworm. The leaves are used for fevers, as well as menstrual and digestion problems.

- In Brazil, lemongrass is used to calm nervousness and for stomach disorders.

- In Thailand, lemongrass is widely used to flavor foods.

- Lemongrass, which is highly aromatic, is widely cultivated in the Asian tropics for the essential oil. It is used in perfumery, to fragrance skin care products, and as a flavoring agent in cooking.

Practical Uses

Improves digestion
Balancing to the nervous system; calming, reduces stress; promotes a restful sleep
Vapors help open the sinus and breathing passages
Mood uplifting; reviving; improves alertness
Reduces inflammation and swollen tissues; contracts weak connective tissue, tones the skin
Increases lactation
Repels insects

Documented Properties

Analgesic, Antibacterial, Antidepressant, Antifungal, Antioxidant, Antiseptic, Antispasmodic, Aperitive, Astringent, Calmative, Carminative, Deodorant, Deodorizer, Depurative, Digestive, Disinfectant, Diuretic, Febrifuge, Galactagogue, Insect Repellent, Insecticide, Nervine, Parasiticide, Regulator (*Parasympathetic System*), Reviving, Sedative, Stimulant (*Circulatory System*), Stomachic, Tonic, Tonifying (*Skin*)

Aromatherapy Methods of Use: Application, aroma lamp, diffusor, inhaler, light bulb ring, massage, mist spray

CAUTION: Lemongrass oil can irritate the skin and should either be avoided or used with extra care by people who have sensitive skin. Use small amounts.

LEPTOSPERMUM
(New Zealand Tea Tree)

Botanical Name: *Leptospermum citratum, L. ericoides* (Kanuka), *L. petersonii, L. scoparium* (Manuka)
Family: *Myrtaceae*

The essential oil is obtained from the leaves and branches of the shrub.

History and Information

- Leptospermum is an evergreen shrub native to New Zealand and Australia. The shrub grows to a height of about 10 feet and has red flowers.

- The Maori people of New Zealand have used all parts of this valuable shrub to produce healing remedies.

- When Captain Cook and his crew discovered New Zealand in the 18th century, they used leptospermum leaves to make a tea. As a result, the tree became known as New Zealand tea tree.

Practical Uses

Calming; reduces stress and tension
Helps to breath easier
Mood uplifting, aphrodisiac, euphoric; improves mental clarity
Relieves aches and pains; loosens tight muscles
Deodorant (*L. scoparium* variety)
Disinfectant
Healing to the skin

Documented Properties

Analgesic, Antidepressant, Antifungal, Antiseptic, Disinfectant, Sedative, Vulnerary

Aromatherapy Methods of Use: Application, aroma lamp, bath, inhaler, light bulb ring, massage, mist spray, steam and sauna room

LIME

Botanical Name: *Citrus aurantiifolia, C. limetta*
Family: *Rutaceae*

The essential oil is obtained from the peel of the fruit of the tree.

History and Information

- Lime is an evergreen citrus tree native to Asia. The tree grows to a height of about 10 feet and has fragrant white flowers.

- English sailors were called "limeys" because they added limes to their diets to help prevent scurvy.

Practical Uses

Cooling
Purifying; helps in the reduction of cellulite
Strengthens the nerves; used when there is weakness in the body

Reducess stress
Mood uplifting, refreshing, reviving; improves mental clarity and alertness, sharpens the senses
Disinfectant
Soothes insect bites

Documented Properties

Antibacterial, Antidepressant, Antilithic, Antirheumatic, Antisclerotic, Antiscorbutic, Antiseptic, Antispasmodic, Antitoxic, Antiviral, Aperitif, Astringent, Cooling, Depurative, Disinfectant, Febrifuge, Hemostatic, Hepatic, Insecticide, Refreshing, Restorative, Stimulant (*Digestive and Lymphatic Systems*), Tonic (*Immune System*), Uplifting

Aromatherapy Methods of Use: Application, aroma lamp, bath, diffusor, inhaler, light bulb ring, massage, mist spray

CAUTION: Lime oil can irritate the skin and should either be avoided or used with extra care by people who have sensitive skin. Use small amounts. Lime is phototoxic. Avoid exposure to direct sunlight several hours after applying the oil on the skin.

LINDEN BLOSSOM

Botanical Name: *Tilia europaea, T. vulgaris*
Family: *Tiliaceae*

The absolute/essential oil is obtained from the flowers of the tree.

History and Information

- Linden is native to the northern hemisphere. The tree grows to a height of about 130 feet and has clusters of fragrant white flowers. Linden is also known as lime tree or basswood.

- In Europe, the leaves were brewed to make a tea for relaxation and sleep.

Practical Uses

Calming; reduces stress, promotes a restful sleep

Documented Properties

Antidepressant, Antineuralgic, Antiseptic, Antispasmodic, Antistress, Antitussive, Astringent,

Calmative, Carminative, Cephalic, Decongestant, Detoxifier, Diaphoretic, Diuretic, Emollient, Hypotensor, Nervine, Sedative, Stomachic, Sudorific, Tonic (*Nervous System*)

Aromatherapy Methods of Use: Application, aroma lamp, bath, inhaler, light bulb ring, massage, mist spray

CAUTION: Linden blossom oil should not be used over a prolonged period of time.

LITSEA CUBEBA

Botanical Name: *Litsea citrata, L. cubeba*
Family: *Lauraceae*

The essential oil is obtained from fruit of the tree.

History and Information

- Litsea cubeba is an evergreen tree native to Asia. The tree grows to a height of about 30 feet, and has white flowers that develop into small red or black berries. Litsea cubeba is part of sixty species of trees.

- In Chinese medicine, litsea cubeba is used for chest congestion.

- The properties of litsea cubeba are similar to those of lemongrass oil.

- The oil is mainly produced and extensively used in China. The herb is also known as may-chang.

Practical Uses

Cooling
Improves digestion
Calming, reduces stress; promotes a restful sleep
Mood uplifting, reviving, euphoric; improves mental clarity and alertness
Relieves pain

Documented Properties

Antibacterial, Anticongestive, Antidepressant, Antiinflammatory, Antiseptic, Antistress, Aperitive, Astringent, Bronchodilator, Calmative, Carminative, Deodorant, Deodorizer, Detoxifier, Digestive, Disinfectant, Emollient, Galactagogue, Healing

(*Skin*), Insecticide, Revitalizing, Sedative, Stimulant (*Digestion*), Stomachic, Tonic, Uplifting, Vulnerary

Aromatherapy Methods of Use: Application, aroma lamp, diffusor, inhaler, light bulb ring, massage, mist spray

CAUTION: Litsea cubeba oil can irritate the skin and should either be avoided or used with extra care by people who have sensitive skin. Use small amounts.

LOVAGE

Botanical Name: *Angelica levisticum, Levisticum officinale, Ligusticum levisticum*
Family: *Apiaceae*

The essential oil is obtained from the plant root.

History and Information

- Lovage is native to Europe and is also known as love parsley. The plant grows to a height of about 6 feet, and has large dark green leaves and small green flowers.

- Herbalists recommend various preparations of lovage roots to stimulate urine flow and menstruation.

- In Asian countries, the stems are eaten to strengthen the body's defenses against infection and for the cholera disease.

- The plant and roots are eaten fresh in a salad; the seeds flavor baked goods and cooked dishes.

- The root yields approximately 1% essential oil, and is used extensively in perfumery and as a food flavoring.

Practical Uses

Purifying; helps in the reduction of cellulite
Calming; reduces stress
Helps to breathe easier
Mood uplifting, aphrodisiac, euphoric; improves mental clarity and alertness

Documented Properties

Antibacterial, Antifungal, Antiseptic, Antispasmodic, Aphrodisiac, Carminative, Deodorizer, Depura-

tive, Detoxifier, Diaphoretic, Digestive, Diuretic, Emmenagogue, Expectorant, Febrifuge, Laxative, Parasiticide, Revitalizing, Stimulant (*Digestive System and Kidneys*), Stomachic, Warming

Aromatherapy Methods of Use: Application, aroma lamp, bath, inhaler, light bulb ring, massage, mist spray

CAUTION: Lovage is phototoxic. Avoid exposure to direct sunlight several hours after applying the oil on the skin.

MANDARIN & TANGERINE

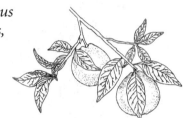

Botanical Name: *Citrus madurensis, C. nobilis, C. reticulata* (Mandarin); *Citrus reticulata* (Tangerine)
Family: *Rutaceae*

The essential oil is obtained from the peel of the fruit.

History and Information

- Mandarin and tangerine are evergreen citrus trees native to Asia. They grow to a height of about 20–25 feet, and have fragrant white flowers that develop into edible fruits.

- The oils are used for flavoring confectionery, beverages, chewing gum, and baked goods. They are also valued in perfumery.

Practical Uses

Cooling
Purifying; helps in the reduction of cellulite
Calming; promotes a restful sleep
Mood uplifting; improves mental clarity, and alertness, sharpens the mind, relieves emotional tension and stress, calms angry and irritable children

Documented Properties

Antidepressant, Antiemetic, Antiseptic, Antispasmodic, Antistress, Antitussive, Aperitive, Astringent, Calmative, Carminative, Cholagogue, Cytophylactic, Decongestant, Depurative, Digestive, Diuretic, Emollient, Hypnotic, Revitalizing, Sedative, Stimulant (*Digestive and Lymphatic*

Systems), Stomachic, Tonic, Tranquilizer, Uplifting

Aromatherapy Methods of Use: Application, aroma lamp, bath, diffusor, inhaler, light bulb ring, massage, mist spray

CAUTION: Mandarin and tangerine oils can irritate the skin and should either be avoided or used with extra care by people who have sensitive skin. Use small amounts. Both oils are phototoxic. Avoid exposure to direct sunlight several hours after applying the oil on the skin.

MARJORAM (Spanish & Sweet)

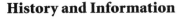

Botanical Name: *Thymus mastichina* (Spanish marjoram); *Majorana hortensis, Origanum majorana* (Sweet marjoram)
Family: *Lamiaceae*

The essential oil is obtained from the flowering tops and leaves of the plant.

History and Information

- Spanish marjoram is native to Spain. The plant grows to a height of about 1 foot.

- Sweet marjoram is a bushy plant native to the Mediterranean area. The plant grows to a height of about 2 feet, and has light green leaves and white or purple flowers.

- Before the discovery of hops, marjoram was said to be used as an essential ingredient in the brewing of beer.

- Marjoram was used by the Egyptians, Greeks, and Romans for common colds and sore throats. The Romans also grew the herb for perfume, digestive aid, to promote menstruation, and heal bruises. The Greeks used it in perfumes and toiletries, for snakebites, and muscle and joint pains.

- The Romans and Greeks used marjoram to crown young couples at weddings.

- Dioscorides, the Greek physician, used marjoram for nervous disorders while Pliny, the Roman herbalist, used it for digestive problems.

- European singers drink marjoram tea to maintain their voices.

- The flowering tops and leaves yield 0.2–0.8% essential oil.

Practical Uses

Warming; improves circulation, dilates the blood vessels
Improves digestion
Relaxing, calms nervous tension, promotes a restful sleep
Vapors open the sinus and breathing passages; especially helpful during colds and nasal congestion
Relieves tense muscles, aches, pains, painful menstruation, inflammation, spasms
Disinfectant

Documented Properties

Analgesic, Anaphrodisiac, Antibacterial, Antifungal, Antioxidant, Antiseptic, Antispasmodic, Antistress, Antitussive, Antiviral, Calmative, Carminative, Cephalic, Cordial, Decongestant, Detoxifier, Diaphoretic, Digestive, Diuretic, Emmenagogue, Expectorant, Febrifuge, Galactagogue, Hypotensor, Laxative, Nervine, Restorative, Sedative, Stomachic, Tonic (*Heart*), Vasodilator (*Arterial*), Vulnerary, Warming

Aromatherapy Methods of Use: Application, aroma lamp, bath, diffusor, inhaler, light bulb ring, massage, mist spray, steam inhalation, steam and sauna room

CAUTION: Due to the relaxing effect of the oil, marjoram should not be used before driving or doing anything that requires full attention. In large amounts, marjoram can be stupefying on the mind.

MASSOIA BARK

Botanical Name: *Cryptocarya massoia*
Family: *Lauraceae*

The essential oil is obtained from the tree bark.

History and Information

- Massoia belongs to a species of two hundred evergreen trees and shrubs that thrive in tropical and subtropical regions of South America, Asia, and the southern part of Africa. The tree has leathery leaves and small flowers.

Practical Uses

Warming; improves circulation
Calming, relaxing
Mood uplifting, aphrodisiac, euphoric, reviving; improves mental clarity and concentration; heightens the senses

Aromatherapy Methods of Use: Application, aroma lamp, diffusor, light bulb ring, inhaler, massage, mist spray

CAUTION: Massoia bark oil can irritate the skin and should be used with extra care. People with sensitive skin should avoid using the oil.

MASTIC

Botanical Name: *Pistacia lentiscus*
Family: *Anacardiaceae*

The resin/essential oil is obtained from the tree bark.

History and Information

- Mastic is an evergreen tree native to the Mediterranean area. The small tree grows to a height of about 10 feet, and has clusters of green fragrant flowers and red to black berries.

- The ancient people chewed on the twigs and bark to strengthen their gums and teeth. This is the origin of the word "masticate." Today, the Turks still chew mastic to sweeten their breaths and keep their gums healthy.

- The Egyptians burned the resin for incense.

- The resin and oil have similar properties to terebinth. The resin is used in baked goods, for halitosis, in varnishes, and to fill dental cavities. Mastic is also known as lentisque oil.

Practical Uses

Vapors open the sinus and breathing passages
Disinfectant

Documented Properties

Antiseptic, Antispasmodic, Astringent, Diuretic, Expectorant, Stimulant

Aromatherapy Methods of Use: Application, inhaler, massage, mist spray, steam inhalation, steam and sauna room

MELISSA (Lemon Balm)

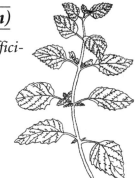

Botanical Name: *Melissa officinalis*
Family: *Lamiaceae*

The essential oil is obtained from the leaves of the plant.

History and Information

- Melissa is native to Europe and the Mediterranean region. The plant grows to a height of about 1–3 feet, and has clusters of small light-blue, yellow, or white flowers.

- The ancient Greeks placed the twigs of melissa in beehives to attract bees.

- Melissa became so popular as a remedy for nervousness and anxiety that Emperor Charlemagne ordered the herb grown in all of his gardens to guarantee an adequate supply.

- The Arabs introduced melissa as a remedy for depression and anxiety, and believed it was good for heart disorders. Avicenna, an Arab physician of the 11th century, recognized the benefits of the herb and used it as an antidote for melancholy.

- In the Middle Ages, herbalists greatly expanded on earlier uses of melissa and recommended it for insomnia, pain, digestive problems, and menstrual cramps. Melissa became known as a cure-all. The herb was also strewn around the house to provide a clean and festive atmosphere.

- Paracelsus, a Swiss physician of the 16th century, highly valued melissa for its ability to revive and rejuvenate the body and uplift the mood.

- Charles V, the king of France, drank lemon balm tea daily to maintain good health. The popularity of the tea was so widespread that it became known as the "tea of France."

- In Germany, the herb is widely used as a tranquilizer. It is also an active ingredient in Lomaherpan Creme, an ointment applied to cold sores and genital herpes.

- Melissa yields a minute quantity of essential oil. Litsea cubeba, lemongrass, and citronella are often blended with or added to melissa and then sold falsely as true melissa oil.

Practical Uses

Calming, relieves nervousness and nervous conditions such as stress, tension and anxiety; promotes a restful sleep
Mood uplifting
Relieves aches, pains, and menstrual pain

Documented Properties

Analgesic, Antibacterial, Anticonvulsive, Antidepressant, Anti-inflammatory, Antioxidant, Antiputrid, Antiseptic, Antispasmodic, Antistress, Antiviral, Aperitive, Calmative, Carminative, Cephalic, Choleretic, Cordial, Cytophylactic, Diaphoretic, Digestive, Emmenagogue, Febrifuge, Galactagogue, Hypotensor, Insect Repellent, Nervine, Sedative, Stomachic, Tonic, Uplifting, Vermifuge, Vulnerary

Aromatherapy Methods of Use: Application, aroma lamp, diffusor, inhaler, light bulb ring, massage, mist spray

CAUTION: Melissa oil can irritate the skin and should either be avoided or used with extra care by people who have sensitive skin. Use small amounts.

MIMOSA

Botanical Name: *Acacia dealbata, A. decurrens*
Family: *Mimosaceae*

The absolute/essential oil is obtained from the flowers of the tree.

History and Information

- Mimosa is native to Australia. The tree grows to a height of about 40–65 feet, and has small feathery leaves and clusters of small yellow fragrant flowers. The tree thrives in dry climates by storing a large quantity of water in the roots. Mimosa is one of the many varieties of the acacia tree.

- The tree is prized for gum arabic, which is secreted from the branches.

- The tree pods are a favorite food of elephants.

Practical Uses

Mood uplifting

Documented Properties

Antidepressant, Anti-inflammatory, Antiseptic, Astringent, Moisturizer (*Skin*), Uplifting

Aromatherapy Methods of Use: Application, aroma lamp, fragrancing, light bulb ring, massage, mist spray

MONARDA

Botanical Name: *Monarda fistulosa*
Family: *Lamiaceae*

The essential oil is obtained from the whole plant.

History and Information

- Monarda is a bushy plant native to the United States. The plant grows to a height of about 4 feet and has whorls of lavender-colored flowers. The entire plant smells similar to citrus.

- American Indians and early American settlers made a tea from the plant for fevers, colds, sore throats, and congestion. They also used monarda to flavor foods.

- The herb was popular during the Boston Tea Party because it was used as a substitute for "black tea."

Practical Uses

Calming, relaxing; reduces stress
Helps the breathing
Mood uplifting; improves mental clarity; brings out feelings

Documented Properties

Antibacterial, Antifungal, Antiseptic, Antiviral, Carminative, Expectorant, Stimulant, Tonic

Aromatherapy Methods of Use: Application, aroma lamp, diffusor, inhaler, light bulb ring, massage, mist spray

CAUTION: Monarda oil can irritate the skin and should either be avoided or used with extra care by people who have sensitive skin. Use small amounts.

MUGWORT (Armoise)

Botanical Name: *Artemisia vulgaris*
Family: *Asteraceae*

The essential oil is obtained from the whole plant.

History and Information

- Mugwort is native to Asia. The bushy plant grows to a height of about 2–8 feet, and has small reddish, yellow, or white flowers.

- Europeans stuffed mugwort into their pillows to inhale all night because they believed that it helped them dream vividly.

- Oriental medicine uses the herb to treat malaria and anemia. In China, a compress of mugwort is used to facilitate childbirth.

- American Indians used the leaves for respiratory congestion, digestive problems, and joint and muscle pains.

- Mugwort is known to regulate the female cycles, and is referred to as a magical plant for its ability to increase one's psychic powers.

- In Europe the herb is added to flavor foods.

Practical Uses

Calming
Helps one to dream
Relieves menstrual cramps

Documented Properties

Abortifacient, Analgesic, Anthelmintic, Anti-inflammatory, Antirheumatic, Antispasmodic, Aperitif, Aperitive, Carminative, Cholagogue, Diaphoretic, Digestive, Diuretic, Emmenagogue, Febrifuge, Insect Repellent, Nervine, Purgative (*Mild*), Regulator (*Menstrual Cycle*), Sedative, Stimulant (*Uterine*), Sudorific, Tonic (*Uterine*), Vermifuge

CAUTION: Mugwort oil contains a toxic component called thujone, which can interfere with the brain and nervous system functions.

MYRRH

Botanical Name: *Balsamodendrom myrrha, Commiphora myrrha*
Family: *Burseraceae*

The resin/essential oil is obtained from the bark of the tree.

History and Information

- Myrrh is native to Africa and Asia. The tree grows to a height of about 9 feet and has yellow-red flowers.

- In the ancient world, myrrh was highly prized and more widely used than any other aromatic oil in perfumes, anointing oils, incense, ointments, medicines, and for embalming purposes.

- The Egyptians believed that the fragrant odor pleased the gods and, therefore, burned the oil during religious ceremonies. The Ebers Papyrus, dated 1550 B.C., contains information on the use of myrrh for facial masks.

- The Greeks used the resin on wounded soldiers to promote healing.

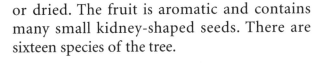

- Myrrh has been used throughout history to maintain healthy teeth and gums.

- The bark contains approximately 8% essential oil.

Practical Uses

Cooling
Calming; promotes a restful sleep
Mood uplifting; helpful for meditation
Soothes inflamed tissue
Used as a fixative to hold the scent of a fragrance
Healing to the skin

Documented Properties

Analgesic, Antidiabetic, Antifungal, Anti-inflammatory, Antiputrid, Antiseptic (*Strong*) (*Infected Gums*), Antispasmodic, Antitussive, Aperitive, Astringent, Balsamic, Carminative, Cicatrizant, Cooling, Deodorant, Depurative, Disinfectant, Diuretic, Drying, Emmenagogue, Expectorant, Fixative, Healing (*Traumatic Injuries*), Hemostatic, Invigorating (*Immune System*), Moisturizer, Pectoral, Rejuvenator (*Skin Cells*), Revitalizing (*Skin*), Sedative, Stimulant (*Digestive System*), Stomachic, Sudorific, Tonic (*Stomach*), Tonifying (*Cleanses and Tightens the Skin*), Vulnerary

Aromatherapy Methods of Use: Application, aroma lamp, bath, inhaler, light bulb ring, massage, mist spray

MYRTLE

Botanical Name: *Myrtus communis*
Family: *Myrtaceae*

The essential oil is obtained from the leaves, twigs, and flowering tops of the shrub.

History and Information

- Myrtle is an evergreen shrub native to Europe and Asia. The plant grows to a height of about 10–18 feet, and has scented leaves and small aromatic white blossoms. The flowers develop into bluish black berries that are edible fresh or dried. The fruit is aromatic and contains many small kidney-shaped seeds. There are sixteen species of the tree.

- The ancient Egyptians and, later, Dioscorides, the Greek physician, macerated myrtle leaves to make a wine for respiratory and bladder afflictions.

- Greek and Roman folklore claimed that tea made from myrtle had the virtue of preserving love and youth. They also used myrtle for its tonic and astringent effect on the skin.

- In Great Britain, it was customary to have myrtle sprigs in the bridal bouquets and for the bridesmaid to plant the sprigs. This connection with weddings has associated myrtle as a symbol of love.

- The branches, twigs, leaves, and berries are used to flavor foods and repel insects. The oil is used in cosmetics and perfumes; the leaves are added to potpourri.

Practical Uses

Calming
Vapors open sinus and breathing passages
Mood uplifting, refreshing; helpful for meditation
Relieves pain

Documented Properties

Antibacterial, Antifungal, Antiseptic, Astringent, Balsamic, Carminative, Expectorant, Hemostatic, Nervine, Parasiticide, Sedative, Tonic (*Skin*)

Aromatherapy Methods of Use: Application, aroma lamp, bath, diffusor, inhaler, light bulb ring, massage, mist spray, steam inhalation, steam and sauna room

NEROLI

Botanical Name: *Citrus aurantium*
Family: *Rutaceae*

The essential oil is obtained from the blossoms of the tree.

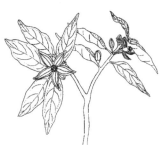

History and Information

- The oil of neroli is produced from the fragrant white blossoms of the bitter orange tree. Bitter orange is an evergreen citrus tree native to Asia.

- Neroli was named in 1680 when the princess of Nerole perfumed her gloves, stationery, shawls, and her bathwater with the scent. For centuries, neroli has been added to cosmetic preparations, colognes, and perfumes.

- Neroli is often adulterated with the essential oil of petitgrain, which has similar properties and is relatively inexpensive.

Practical Uses

Soothes the intestines
Calms nervous tension, relaxes hyperactive children; promotes a restful sleep
Mood uplifting; boosts confidence, helps to face emotional fear
Helps to relieve menstrual discomfort

Documented Properties

Analgesic, Antibacterial, Antidepressant, Antifungal, Antiseptic, Antispasmodic, Antistress, Aphrodisiac, Astringent, Blood Purifier, Calmative, Carminative, Cicatrizant, Cordial, Cytophylactic, Deodorant, Digestive, Emollient, Euphoriant, Hypnotic, Hypotensor, Regenerator (*Skin Cells*), Sedative, Tonic, Tranquilizer, Uplifting

Aromatherapy Methods of Use: Application, aroma lamp, bath, inhaler, light bulb ring, massage, mist spray

NIAOULI

Botanical Name: *Melaleuca quinquenervia, M. viridiflora*
Family: *Myrtaceae*

The essential oil is obtained from the leaves and twigs of the bush.

History and Information

- Niaouli is an evergreen bush with yellow flowers and is native to Australia.

- The oil of niaouli is also known as gomenol oil.

Practical Uses

Vapors open sinus and breathing passages
Relieves aches and pains

Documented Properties

Analgesic, Anthelmintic, Antibacterial, Antirheumatic, Antiseptic, Antispasmodic, Balsamic, Cicatrizant, Decongestant, Diaphoretic, Expectorant, Febrifuge, Insecticide, Regenerator (*Skin Tissue*), Reviving, Stimulant (*Circulation to the Tissues*), Tonic (*Respiratory System*), Vermifuge, Vulnerary

Aromatherapy Methods of Use: Application, aroma lamp, bath, diffusor, inhaler, light bulb ring, massage, mist spray, steam inhalation, steam and sauna room

NUTMEG

Botanical Name: *Myristica aromata, M. fragrans, M. officinalis*
Family: *Myristicaceae*

The essential oil is obtained from the seeds of the tree.

History and Information

- Nutmeg is an evergreen tree native to the Molucca Islands. The tree grows to a height of about 60–80 feet and has small yellow flowers that develop into yellow fruits. The flowers of the female tree bear fruit after being pollinated from flowers of the male tree. The leaves are large and fragrant.

- Hindu practitioners in India have used nutmeg since early times. The herb was used for pain, bad breath, and intestinal disorders.

- The herb was recommended in the Arabian writings as an aphrodisiac, and to treat urinary and digestive disorders.

- The kernel contains approximately 10% essential oil.

Practical Uses

Slightly warming
Improves digestion
Calming and promotes a restful sleep in small amounts
Mood uplifting, reviving; mental stimulant, improves mental clarity and alertness; helps one to dream
Loosens tight muscles; relieves aches, pains, sore muscles and menstrual pains

Documented Properties

Analgesic, Antibacterial, Antiemetic, Antioxidant, Antirheumatic, Antiseptic, Antispasmodic, Aperitive, Aphrodisiac, Astringent, Calmative, Cardiac, Carminative, Digestive, Emmenagogue, Estrogenic, Expectorant, Invigorating, Laxative, Reviving, Sedative, Stimulant (*Circulatory System*), Stomachic, Tonic, Uplifting, Warming

Aromatherapy Methods of Use: Application, aroma lamp, bath, diffusor, inhaler, light bulb ring, massage, mist spray

CAUTION: Nutmeg oil is toxic if used in large amounts and can cause a stupefying effect.

ORANGE, TANGELO & TEMPLE ORANGE

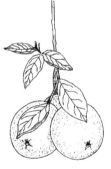

Botanical Name: *Citrus aurantium* (Bitter orange); *Citrus reticulata* (Temple orange); *Citrus sinensis* (Sweet orange); *Citrus tangelo* (Tangelo)
Family: *Rutaceae*

The essential oil is obtained from the peel of the fruit.

History and Information

- Orange, tangelo, and temple orange are evergreen citrus trees native to Asia. The trees grow to a height of about 20–30 feet and have fragrant white flowers that develop into edible citrus fruit.

- The tangelo tree was first produced in 1897 by the United States Agriculture Department. The tangelo fruit is a hybrid cross between a tangerine and a grapefruit.

- Temple orange is a cross between a tangerine and an orange hybrid. The tree was propagated in 1917 in Florida and named after William Chace Temple, who was a prominent person in the citrus field.

- In Chinese folk medicine, the dried orange fruit was used as a remedy for swelling in the stomach and indigestion.

- Oranges are one of the most popular of all the fruits. The seeds yield an oil that is used for cooking, and as an ingredient in soaps and plastics. The oil from the rind is used in food flavorings, cosmetics, and perfumes, and is added to wood-care products to protect against insect damage.

Practical Uses

Cooling
Purifying; helps in the reduction of cellulite
Calming, reduces stress; promotes a restful sleep
Mood uplifting; improves mental clarity and alertness; relieves emotional tension and stress, calms angry and irritable children
Relieves spasms

Documented Properties

Antibacterial, Anticoagulant, Antidepressant, Antiemetic, Antifungal, Anti-inflammatory, Antipyorrhea, Antiscorbutic, Antiseptic, Antispasmodic, Antistress, Antitoxic, Antitussive, Antiviral, Aperitif, Aperitive, Astringent, Calmative, Carminative, Cholagogue, Choleretic, Depurative, Digestive, Disinfectant, Diuretic, Expectorant, Febrifuge, Hemostatic, Hepatic, Hypotensor, Hypnotic, Laxative, Nervine, Refreshing, Sedative, Stimulant (*Digestive and Lymphatic Systems*), Stomachic, Tonic, Vasoconstrictor, Vulnerary

Aromatherapy Methods of Use: Application, aroma lamp, bath, diffusor, inhaler, light bulb ring, massage, mist spray

CAUTION: Orange, tangelo, and temple orange oils can irritate the skin and should either be avoided or used with extra care by people who have sensitive skin. Use small amounts. These oils are phototoxic. Avoid exposure to direct sunlight several hours after applying the oil on the skin.

OREGANO

Botanical Name: *Origanum vulgare*
Family: *Lamiaceae*

The essential oil is obtained from the flowering plant.

History and Information

- Oregano is native to Europe and America. The plant grows to a height of about 1–2 feet, and has dark green leaves and purple buds that blossom into white, pink, or lilac-colored flowers. The entire plant is aromatic. There are about twenty species of oregano.

- The Greeks used oregano to heal wounds, and placed the leaves on sore and aching muscles to relieve their discomfort. Dioscorides, the Greek physician, used oregano for poisonous animal bites.

- Pliny, the Roman herbalist, recommended oregano for poisonous spider bites and to improve digestion.

- During the Middle Ages, oregano was used by herbalists for improving digestion, eyesight, and for poisonous bites.

- Modern herbalists use oregano to aid digestion, headaches, coughs, promote menstruation, and prevent sea sickness.

- The common name of the plant is wild marjoram. The essential oil is one of the most antiseptic of all the oils and is also known as origanum oil.

Practical Uses

Heating; improves circulation
Improves digestion
Purifying; helps in the reduction of cellulite
Vapors open the sinus and breathing passages
Mood uplifting; improves mental clarity and alertness
Relieves muscle aches and pains
Increases physical endurance and energy
Increases perspiration
Disinfectant
Repels insects

Documented Properties

Analgesic, Anaphrodisiac, Anthelmintic, Antibacterial, Antifungal, Anti-inflammatory, Antirheumatic, Antiseptic, Antispasmodic, Antitoxic, Antiviral, Aperitif, Aperitive, Balsamic, Carminative, Cholagogue, Choleretic, Cytophylactic, Diaphoretic, Disinfectant, Diuretic, Emmenagogue, Expectorant, Febrifuge, Hepatic, Hypnotic, Laxative, Parasiticide, Rubefacient, Stimulant (*Nerves*), Stomachic, Sudorific, Tonic, Vulnerary, Warming

Aromatherapy Methods of Use: Application, aroma lamp, diffusor, inhaler, light bulb ring, massage, mist spray

CAUTION: Oregano oil can irritate the skin and should either be avoided or used with extra care by people who have sensitive skin. Use small amounts.

ORRIS ROOT

Botanical Name: *Iris florentina, I. pallida*
Family: *Iridaceae*

The concrete/absolute/essential oil/powder is obtained from the root of the plant.

History and Information

- Orris is native to the Mediterranean area. The plant grows to a height of about 2½ feet, and has sword-like leaves and large scented flowers ranging in various colors, depending on the variety.

- The Egyptians, Greeks, and Romans used orris root for perfume. The plant was found depicted on the walls of an Egyptian temple dated about 1500 B.C.

- Orris root was used as a dry shampoo in the 18th century, and up until the 20th century it was also used as a face powder.

- The root requires a 3-year growing period before it can be harvested; it is then left to dry for 2–3 years until it acquires a scent similar to violets.

- The oil is extensively used to perfume soaps, powders, toothpastes, and sweets.

Documented Properties

Analgesic, Anthelmintic, Antidiarrhoeic, Diuretic, Expectorant, Fixative, Purgative, Stomachic

CAUTION: Orris root is toxic.

OSMANTHUS

Botanical Name: *Osmanthus fragrans*
Family: *Oleaceae*

The absolute/essential oil is obtained from the flowers of the tree.

History and Information

- Osmanthus is an evergreen tree native to Asia and the United States. The tree has leathery leaves and clusters of white or yellow flowers with a jasmine-like scent. The flowers develop into black, blue, or violet-colored oval fruits. Osmanthus belongs to the olive family.

- In China, osmanthus flowers are added to foods and beverages, and the oil is used in expensive perfumes.

Practical Uses

Calming; reduces stress

Documented Properties

Antidepressant, Calmative, Sedative

Aromatherapy Methods of Use: Application, massage

PALMAROSA

Botanical Name: *Andronpogon martinii, Cymbopogon martinii* var. *motia*
Family: *Poaceae*

The essential oil is obtained from the plant, which is a grass.

History and Information

- Palmarosa is a fragrant grass native to Asia. The plant grows to a height of about 9 feet and has clusters of flowers that turn red when they mature.

- The expensive oil of rose is often adulterated with palmarosa, which is cheaper in price.

- Palmarosa is also known as rosha or rusha. The oil is widely used in perfumery and cosmetology.

Practical Uses

Warming; improves circulation
Calming; reduces stress
Mood uplifting, refreshing
Reduces aches, pains, and inflammation
Moisturizing and regenerating to the skin

Documented Properties

Antibacterial, Antifungal, Antiseptic, Antistress, Antiviral, Aperitive, Calmative, Cicatrizant, Cytophylactic, Digestive, Emollient, Febrifuge, Moisturizer, Nervine, Refreshing, Regenerator (*Skin Cells*), Stimulant (*Circulatory and Digestive Systems*), Tonic, Uplifting, Vermifuge

Aromatherapy Methods of Use: Application, aroma lamp, bath, diffusor, inhaler, light bulb ring, massage, mist spray

PARSLEY

Botanical Name: *Apium petroselinum, Carum petroselinum, Petroselinum hortense, P. sativum*
Family: *Apiaceae*

The essential oil is obtained from the seeds of the plant.

History and Information

- Parsley is native to the Mediterranean area and Africa. The plant grows to a height of about 3 feet and has green-yellow flowers.

- Theophrastus, the father of botany, claimed parsley benefited the heart.

- The Greeks used parsley to crown victors at their games and decorate tombs.

- The Romans were the first people to use parsley for food and to counter bad odors.

- Emperor Charlemagne ordered parsley grown in his imperial gardens to insure that he had an adequate supply for each meal.

- Female peasants in the Mediterranean area used parsley leaves to relieve breast soreness and curtail lactation of nursing mothers.

- Parsley tea was used in World War I for kidney problems caused by dysentery.

- The herb was used in large doses by pregnant women to abort the fetus. In France, apiol, a constituent of parsley, was used for contraception before birth control pills were available. Apiol is also used in South America as a contraceptive. The oil is a powerful uterine stimulant and must be avoided during pregnancy.

- The root has been used to reduce thyroid activity.

- Parsley seeds have been known to be deadly to birds.

- The parsley plant contains a rich source of protein, potassium, calcium, and vitamin C, which are valuable in the mending of bones, strengthening blood vessels, and keeping the skin and muscles healthy. A deficiency of vitamin C is known to result in easy bruising of the skin and slow healing of broken bones. The seeds yield 3–6% essential oil and the leaves yield 0.25%.

Practical Uses

Improves digestion
Calms the nerves
Eliminates excess water from the body

Documented Properties

Abortifacient, Antianemia, Antigalactagogue, Anti-inflammatory, Antilithic, Antirheumatic, Antiseptic, Antispasmodic, Aperient, Aperitive (*In Small Amounts*), Aphrodisiac, Blood Builder, Blood Purifier, Calmative, Carminative, Cooling, Depurative, Digestive, Diuretic (*Strong*), Emmenagogue (*Strong*), Estrogenic, Expectorant, Febrifuge, Hepatic, Insect Repellent, Laxative, Ophthalmic, Parasiticide (*Intestinal*), Sedative, Stimulant (*Kidneys; Uterine Contractions*), Stomachic, Tonic (*Female Reproductive and Circulatory System*), Vasodilator, Vermifuge

Aromatherapy Methods of Use: Application, aroma lamp, inhaler, light bulb ring, massage, mist spray

CAUTION: Due to the toxicity of the oil, use small amounts. Parsley oil can irritate the skin and should either be avoided or used with extra care by people who have sensitive skin. Parsley is phototoxic. Avoid exposure to direct sunlight several hours after applying the oil on the skin.

PATCHOULI

Botanical Name: *Pogostemon cablin, P. patchouli*
Family: *Lamiaceae*

The essential oil is obtained from the leaves of the plant.

History and Information

- Patchouli is native to Asia. The plant grows to a height of about 3 feet, and has whorls of light purple or lavender flowers. Patchouli requires full sun to bring out its fragrance.

- The Arabs used patchouli to repel fleas and lice from their bedding.

- In the Philippines, an infusion of the leaves is taken for menstrual cramps.

- The leaves yield approximately 2.5% essential oil.

Practical Uses

Nerve stimulant; prevents sleep
Mood uplifting, euphoric, aphrodisiac
Repels insects
Healing to the skin

Documented Properties

Alterative, Antibacterial, Analgesic, Antidepressant, Antiemetic, Antifungal, Anti-inflammatory, Antiphlogistic, Antiseptic, Antistress, Antitoxic, Antiviral, Aphrodisiac, Astringent (*Strong*), Calmative, Carminative, Cicatrizant (*Strong*), Cytophylactic, Decongestant, Deodorant, Diaphoretic, Digestive, Diuretic, Febrifuge, Fixative, Insect Repellent, Insecticide, Laxative, Nervine, Parasiticide, Regenerator (*Skin Tissue*), Sedative (*Large Amounts*), Stimulant (*Small Amounts*) (*Nerves*), Stomachic, Tonic (*Uterus*)

Aromatherapy Methods of Use: Application, aroma lamp, bath, inhaler, light bulb ring, massage, mist spray

PENNYROYAL

Botanical Name: *Mentha pulegium*
Family: *Lamiaceae*

The essential oil is obtained from the flowering plant.

History and Information

- Pennyroyal is native to England. The plant grows to a height of about 1 foot and has purple aromatic flowers.

- The Romans used the leaves to repel fleas and insects.

- During medieval times, the plant was strewn throughout households to freshen the air and provide a pleasant fragrance.

- Pennyroyal was used by sailors in the 16th century to purify drinking water.

- In the 19th century, the herb was commonly used in folk medicine to promote perspiration during the onset of a cold and stimulate menstruation; pennyroyal tea was given to babies to help with stomach problems.

- From 1831 through 1916, the herb was listed in the United States pharmacopoeia as a carminative, emmenagogue, and stimulant.

Practical Uses

Repels insects

Documented Properties

Abortifacient, Analgesic, Antipruritic, Antiseptic, Antispasmodic, Blood Purifier, Carminative, Diaphoretic, Digestive, Emmenagogue, Expectorant, Febrifuge, Insect Repellent, Sedative (*Mild*), Stimulant (*Circulatory System*), Stomachic, Warming

CAUTION: Pennyroyal oil is toxic.

PEPPER (Black)

Botanical Name: *Piper nigrum*
Family: *Piperaceae*

The essential oil is obtained from the fruits of the plant.

History and Information

- Black pepper is a tropical climbing vine native to India. The plant grows to a height of about 10 feet and has clusters of small white flowers. As the berries ripen, they turn from green to orange to red. After the berries are picked, they are left in the sun to dry, which turns their color to black.

- Black pepper is one of the oldest known spices used in India, ancient Greece, and Rome for thousands of years.

- Hippocrates claimed that pepper assisted digestion.

- Throughout medieval Europe, this precious spice was commonly traded ounce for ounce for gold. During the Middle Ages and the siege of Rome in 400 A.D., the spice was used as currency.

- During the Middle Ages, pepper was the most important commodity traded between India and Europe. Rents and taxes were frequently paid with pepper.

- Workers unloading black pepper from ships were forbidden to wear clothes with pockets in order to insure that they did not steal the valuable peppercorns.

- In India, pepper is used for liver problems and hemorrhoids.

- The fruits yield approximately 3% essential oil. Pepper is one of the most consumed spices throughout the world. White pepper is produced by removing the dark, outer skin of the black pepper, which gives it a milder taste. Ground-up peppercorns lose their spicy flavor rapidly after being ground.

Practical Uses

Warming; increases circulation
Improves digestion in small amounts
Improves mental clarity; stimulating, reviving
Loosens tight muscles
Improves the benefits of other oils that are used together with black pepper

Documented Properties

Analgesic, Antibacterial, Anticholeric, Anticonvulsive, Antidote, Antiemetic, Antiseptic, Antispasmodic, Antitoxic, Antitussive, Aperitive, Aphrodisiac, Cardiac, Carminative, Detoxifier, Diaphoretic, Digestive, Diuretic, Drying, Expectorant, Febrifuge, Heating, Insect Repellent, Insecticide, Laxative, Rubefacient, Sedative, Stimulant (*Circulation; Kidneys*), Stomachic, Tonic, Tonifying (*Muscles*), Vasodilator

Aromatherapy Methods of Use: Application, massage, mist spray

CAUTION: Black pepper oil can irritate the skin and should either be avoided or used with extra care by people who have sensitive skin. Use small amounts.

PEPPERMINT

Botanical Name:
Mentha piperita
Family: *Lamiaceae*

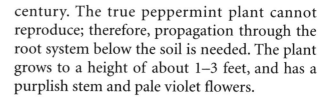

The essential oil is obtained from the whole plant.

History and Information

- Peppermint is a cross between a number of wild mints and has been known since the 17th century. The true peppermint plant cannot reproduce; therefore, propagation through the root system below the soil is needed. The plant grows to a height of about 1–3 feet, and has a purplish stem and pale violet flowers.

- Peppermint capsules are used in Europe for irritated bowels. The extract is effective against herpes simplex and other viral organisms. The oil stops spasms of smooth muscles. It is also an important ingredient in many personal hygiene products, such as aftershave lotions, colognes, and dental toothpastes.

- The leaves yield 0.1–0.8% essential oil.

Practical Uses

Cooling
Improves digestion; increases appetite; relieves flatulence and nausea, freshens bad breath, sweetens the intestines
Vapors open sinus and breathing passages
Mood uplifting especially to people who have a slow metabolism; refreshing, reviving, aphrodisiac; stimulates the brain, nerves, and metabolism; increases mental clarity, alertness, and the ability to concentrate, sharpens the senses; encourages communication; helps to revive a person from a fainting spell or shock
Increases physical strength and endurance
Relieves pain, inflammation, menstrual pain, and cramps
Reduces lactation
Repels insects, kills parasites
Soothes itching skin

Documented Properties

Alterative (*Mild*), Analgesic, Anesthetic, Antibacterial, Anticonvulsive, Antidepressant, Antidiarrhoeic, Antigalactagogue, Anti-inflammatory, Antineuralgic, Antiphlogistic, Antipruritic, Antiseptic, Antispasmodic (*Digestive System*), Antitoxic (*Gastrointestinal Poisoning*), Antitussive, Antiviral, Aperitive, Aphrodisiac, Astringent, Carminative, Cephalic, Cholagogue, Cordial, Decongestant, Depurative, Digestive, Emmenagogue, Expectorant, Febrifuge, Hepatic, Insect Repellent, Invigorating, Nervine, Parasiticide,

Refreshing, Refrigerant, Restorative, Stimulant (*Nervous System*), Stomachic, Sudorific, Tonic (*Heart*), Uplifting, Vasoconstrictor, Vermifuge

Aromatherapy Methods of Use: Application, aroma lamp, diffusor, inhaler, light bulb ring, massage, mist spray, steam inhalation, steam and sauna room

CAUTION: Peppermint oil can irritate the skin and should either be avoided or used with extra care by people who have sensitive skin. Use small amounts. Avoid using before bedtime since the oil can overstimulate the nervous system.

PERU BALSAM

Botanical Name: *Myrosperum pereira, Myroxylon pereirae, Toluifera pereira*
Family: *Fabaceae*

The resin/essential oil is obtained from the bark of the tree.

History and Information

- Peru balsam is a slow-growing evergreen tree native to Central America. The tree grows to a height of about 60–120 feet and has fragrant flowers. Peru balsam is also known as black balsam or Indian balsam.

- The tree thrives in El Salvador. However, the resin was exported to Europe from ports in Peru and, thus, derived the name Peru balsam.

- In the 17th century, the Germans used Peru balsam in their medicine and, thereafter, its use spread universally.

- The Indians in Central and South America consider the Peru bark to be effective to stop bleeding and promote healing. The leaves are used as a diuretic and to expel parasitic worms. In addition, the dried fruits are used to relieve itching, and the resin is used to heal skin bruises and cuts.

- In China, Peru balsam is used as a fragrance and fixative in oriental-type perfumes and cosmetics.

- In the United States, the resin is an ingredient in dental cements, suppositories (to relieve itching of hemorrhoids), as a flavor additive, fragrance, and fungicide. It is also used extensively in topical preparations to heal skin tissue.

- An aromatic, dark brown resin begins to flow when the tree trunk is wounded. The fruits also yield a balsam, which is extracted.

Practical Uses

Warming; increases circulation
Purifying
Calming, reduces stress; promotes a restful sleep
Mood uplifting; helpful for meditation
Loosens tight muscles; helps to move stagnant blood
Used as a fixative to hold a scent of a fragrance
Healing to the skin; improves poor skin conditions

Documented Properties

Antifungal, Anti-inflammatory, Antipruritic, Antiseptic, Balsamic, Emollient, Expectorant, Healing, Parasiticide (*Skin*), Rubefacient, Stimulant, Vulnerary

Aromatherapy Methods of Use: Application, aroma lamp, light bulb ring, inhaler, massage, mist spray

CAUTION: Peru balsam oil can irritate the skin and should either be avoided or used with extra care by people who have sensitive skin. Use small amounts.

PETITGRAIN

Botanical Name: *Citrus bigaradia*
Family: *Rutaceae*

The essential oil is obtained from the leaves and twigs of the tree.

History and Information

- Petitgrain oil is derived from the leaves and twigs of the orange, lemon, or tangerine tree. The citrus evergreen trees are native to Asia.

● The oil is widely used in perfumery.

Practical Uses

Cooling
Calms the nerves, relieves anxiety, tension and mental stress, promotes a restful sleep
Mood uplifting; improves mental clarity and alertness; helpful for meditation
Soothes inflamed and irritated skin tissue

Documented Properties

Antidepressant, Antiseptic, Antispasmodic, Anti-stress, Astringent, Calmative, Deodorant, Digestive, Fixative, Nervine, Refreshing, Sedative, Stimulant (*Digestive System*), Stomachic, Tonic, Uplifting

Aromatherapy Methods of Use: Application, aroma lamp, bath, diffusor, inhaler, light bulb ring, massage, mist spray

PINE

Botanical Name: *Pinus sylvestris*
Family: *Pinaceae*

The essential oil is obtained from the needles and small branches of the tree.

History and Information

● Pine is an evergreen tree native to Asia and Europe. The tree grows to a height about 115–130 feet and has greenish-blue needle-like leaves. There are ninety species of the trees in the pine family. It is estimated that a pine can live to 1200 years.

● The American Indians used pine needles to prevent scurvy, and the bark and berries for rheumatism, broken bones, bruises, sores, inflammation, colds, coughs, lung ailments, headaches, and to fight infection.

● The major uses of the pine tree are: wood for construction, furniture, boats, paper products, turpentine, pine oil, and pine nuts for food. Turpentine, the largest produced oil in the United States, is extracted from the lumber by-products of the pine tree.

Practical Uses

Purifying; removes lymphatic deposits from the body; helps in the reduction of cellulite
Vapors open sinus and breathing passages
Mood uplifting, refreshing, reviving; improves mental clarity, alertness, and memory
Lessens pain
Stimulates the adrenal glands; promotes vitality
Disinfectant

Documented Properties

Analgesic, Antibacterial, Antifungal, Antineuralgic, Antiphlogistic, Antirheumatic, Antiseptic (*Strong*), Antiscorbutic, Antispasmodic, Antitussive, Antiviral, Balsamic, Cholagogue, Choleretic, Decongestant, Deodorant, Depurative (*Kidneys*), Disinfectant, Diuretic, Expectorant, Hypertensor, Insecticide, Laxative, Pectoral, Refreshing, Restorative, Reviving, Rubefacient, Stimulant (*Circulatory and Nervous Systems; Adrenal Glands*), Sudorific, Tonic, Vermifuge, Vulnerary

Aromatherapy Methods of Use: Application, aroma lamp, bath, diffusor, inhaler, light bulb ring, massage, mist spray, steam inhalation, steam and sauna room

CAUTION: **Pine oil has a strong diuretic effect on the kidneys and can also irritate the skin. Use small amounts with care.**

RAVENSARA ANISATA (Havozo Bark)

Botanical Name: *Cinnamonum camphora, Ravensara anisata*
Family: *Lauraceae*

The essential oil is obtained from the bark of the tree.

History and Information

● Ravensara is small tree native to Madagascar. There are eighteen species of the tree.

● The seeds, leaves, and bark taste like cloves and are used as a spice known as Madagascar clove nutmeg. The bark is used in making an alcoholic rum drink.

Practical Uses

Warming
Soothes the intestines
Calming; reduces stress, promotes a restful sleep
Vapors open the sinus and breathing passages
Mood uplifting, aphrodisiac, euphoric; improves mental clarity; encourages communication
Relieves aches, pains, and menstrual discomfort; loosens tight muscles

Documented Properties

Antispasmodic, Carminative, Cholagogue, Choleretic, Emmenagogue, Estrogenic, Galactagogue, Stomachic, Tonic

Aromatherapy Methods of Use: Application, aroma lamp, bath, diffusor, inhaler, light bulb ring, massage, mist spray, steam inhalation, steam and sauna room

RAVENSARA AROMATICA

Botanical Name: *Cinnamonum camphora, Ravensara aromatica*
Family: *Lauraceae*

The essential oil is obtained from the leaves of the tree.

History and Information

Please see Ravensara Anisata.

Practical Uses

Calming; reduces stress
Vapors open the sinus and breathing passages
Mood uplifting, refreshing; improves mental clarity
Relieves aches and pains

Documented Properties

Analgesic, Antibacterial, Antiseptic, Antispasmodic, Antitoxic, Antitussive, Antiviral, Carminative, Cholagogue, Choleretic, Expectorant, Febrifuge, Sedative, Tonic

Aromatherapy Methods of Use: Application, aroma lamp, bath, diffusor, inhaler, light bulb ring, massage, mist spray, steam inhalation, steam and sauna room

RHODODENDRON

Botanical Name: *Rhododendron anthopogon*
Family: *Ericaceae*

The essential oil is obtained from the leaves and flowers of the plant.

History and Information

- Rhododendron is native to the northern hemisphere. The plant grows to a height of about 2 feet, and has glossy leaves and white or pink flowers. The plant belongs to a species of 850 trees and shrubs.

Practical Uses

Calming; reduces stress
Vapors help open the sinus and breathing passages
Mood uplifting; improves mental clarity, mentally energizing

Aromatherapy Methods of Use: Application, aroma lamp, bath, diffusor, inhaler, light bulb ring, massage, mist spray, steam inhalation

ROSE

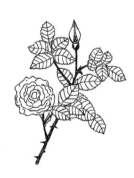

Botanical Name: *Rosa centifolia, R. damascena*
Family: *Rosaceae*

The absolute/essential oil is obtained from the flowers of the bush.

History and Information

- Rose is native to the Mediterranean area. The different varieties of bushes grow to various heights and produce sweet, fragrant flowers.

- Roses have been used throughout history for their appearance, scent, and therapeutic properties. The oil was considered more precious and valuable than gold.

- Hippocrates recommended rose flowers mixed with oil for uterine problems.

- Ayurvedic practitioners used rose petals for skin wounds, inflammations, and also as a laxative.

- The Romans greatly favored the rose and introduced its use to all the people they conquered.

- The Persians were thought to have originated the distillation of rose oil before the Christian era.

- The fragrance symbolizes the love and beauty that was offered to the kings and gods. Cleopatra strewed red rose pedals to a height of 18 inches when she first met Mark Anthony.

- The Persians, Greeks, and Romans bathed their bodies in rose fragrance and used the perfume lavishly during religious ceremonies, burials, and sacrifices.

- Wines and drinks were fragranced with roses by the Persians, Romans, and British.

- Arabic doctors were the first to use rose as a remedy in the form of a jam, while Arabian women used rose as an ingredient in their eye cosmetics.

- American Indians healed mouth sores, fever sores, and blisters with rose. A tea was made from the flowers to strengthen the heart, and to soothe coughs, sore throats, and stomach and liver disorders.

- The most expensive oil is damask rose, which comes from Bulgaria.

Practical Uses

Cooling
Purifying
Calming; reduces stress
Mood uplifting, aphrodisiac; calms emotional shock and grief
Lessens aches, pains, and inflammation
Balances the female hormonal and reproductive system
Regenerates the skin cells; especially beneficial for dry, sensitive, inflamed, red, aging skin

Documented Properties

Antibacterial, Antidepressant, Anti-inflammatory, Antiphlogistic, Antiseptic, Antispasmodic, Antistress, Antiviral, Aperient, Aphrodisiac, Astringent (*Mild*), Calmative, Carminative, Cephalic, Cholagogue, Choleretic, Cicatrizant, Cytophylactic, Depurative, Digestive, Diuretic, Emmenagogue, Emollient, Hemostatic, Hepatic, Laxative, Nervine, Nutritive, Pectoral, Regenerator (*Skin Cells*), Sedative, Stimulant (*Circulatory System*), Stomachic, Tonic (*Nerves*), Tonifying, Uplifting

Aromatherapy Methods of Use: Application, aroma lamp, bath, fragancing, inhaler, light bulb ring, massage, mist spray

ROSEMARY

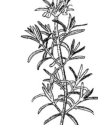

Botanical Name: *Rosmarinus coronarium, R. officinalis*
Family: *Lamiaceae*

The essential oil is obtained from the flowers and leaves of the shrub.

History and Information

- Rosemary is an evergreen shrub native to the Mediterranean region. The bushy plant grows to a height of about 2–6 feet, and has needle-shaped leaves and blue flowers. The entire plant is aromatic.

- Rosemary has long been a symbol of love, loyalty, and eternity. The plant also became known as a symbol of remembrance. Brides wore rosemary wreaths and carried rosemary bouquets to show that they would always remember their families. During funerals, mourners threw fresh rosemary into the grave to signify that the dead would not be forgotten.

- The ancients honored their gods by decorating the statues with the aromatic plant. They also planted rosemary around tombs.

- In ancient Greece, students wore the sprigs of rosemary in their hair while they studied, to strengthen their memory.

- Dioscorides, the Greek physician, recommended rosemary boiled in water as a remedy for jaundice.

- The Arabians claimed rosemary helped the brain and memory.

- Rosemary oil was one of the first essential oils to be distilled, in the year 1330.

- In the Middle Ages, the plant was burned to fumigate sickrooms in order to protect against rampant diseases, and as incense for funeral services. Rosemary was also used in the courts to prevent the spread of jail fever.

- In the 16th century, wealthy families hired perfumers to fragrance their homes with rosemary incense.

- During the plague of 1665, the herb was carried along in the handles of walking sticks and pouches so that the vapors could be inhaled when traveling through infected areas.

- Rosemary oil was recommended by many apothecaries to prevent baldness.

- Gypsies valued the herb for its beneficial effect on their hair and skin.

- During World War II, a mixture of rosemary leaves and juniper berries was burned in the hospitals in France to kill germs.

- The Europeans combine rosemary with white wine as a remedy for poor circulation.

- The plant yields 0.5–1.5% essential oil, which is used in cosmetics, soaps, perfumes, deodorants, and hair tonics.

Practical Uses

Warming; improves circulation
Improves digestion
Purifying; removes cellulite and lymphatic deposits out of the body
Stimulating to the nerves
Vapors open sinus and breathing passages
Mood uplifting to people who tend to have a slower metabolism; stimulates the heart, adrenal glands, metabolism, and all other body functions; refreshing, improves mental clarity, alertness, and the memory
Relieves aches and pains
Disinfectant
Repels insects

Documented Properties

Analgesic, Antidepressant, Antifungal, Antineuralgic, Antioxidant, Antirheumatic, Antiseptic, Antispasmodic, Antitoxic, Antitussive, Aphrodisiac, Astringent, Carminative, Cephalic, Cholagogue, Choleretic, Cicatrizant, Cordial, Cytophylactic, Decongestant (*Liver*), Detoxifier, Diaphoretic, Digestive, Diuretic, Emmenagogue, Expectorant, Hepatic, Hypertensor, Insecticide (*Strong*), Invigorating, Laxative, Nervine, Parasiticide, Pectoral, Rejuvenator (*Skin Cells*), Resolvent, Reviving, Rubefacient, Stimulant (*Adrenal Glands and Nerves*), Stomachic, Sudorific, Tonic, Vulnerary, Warming

Aromatherapy Method of Use: Application, aroma lamp, bath, diffusor, inhaler, light bulb ring, massage, mist spray, steam inhalation, steam and sauna room

CAUTION: Rosemary should not be used by people prone to epileptic seizures.

RUE

Botanical Name: *Ruta graveolens*
Family: *Rutaceae*

The essential oil is obtained from the plant.

History and Information

- Rue is a evergreen plant native to the Mediterranean region. The plant grows to about 3 feet high, and has aromatic leaves and greenish-yellow flowers.

- The Greeks used rue as the main ingredient in a poison antidote.

- The early Romans recognized rue as a very helpful remedy for more than eighty complaints.

- During the first century A.D., Pliny, the Roman herbalist, reported that rue helped improve eyesight.

- Herbalists in the 16th and 17th centuries suggested rue as an antidote for snakebites.

- According to the American Indians, the plant assisted in promoting fertility.

Practical Uses

Lessens pain

Documented Properties

Abortifacient, Anthelmintic, Antidote, Antiseptic, Antispasmodic, Antitoxic, Antitussive, Antiviral, Aperitive, Carminative, Cephalic, Cholagogue, Detoxifier, Diuretic, Emmenagogue, Expectorant, Febrifuge, Insecticide, Nervine, Rubefacient, Sedative, Stimulant (*Digestive System*), Stomachic, Tonic, Vasodilator, Vermifuge

CAUTION: Rue oil is toxic.

SAFFRON

Botanical Name: *Crocus sativus*
Family: *Iridaceae*

The essential oil is obtained from the dried stigma of the plant.

History and Information

- Saffron is native to the Mediterranean. The plant grows to a height of about 1 foot, and has grass-like leaves and fragrant purple flowers.

- Saffron has been known to be used since 1600 B.C.

- Saffron was added to cinnamon and cassia to anoint the Egyptian pharaohs.

- During ancient times, the plant symbolized beauty and youth, and was presented to newlyweds.

- Roman women colored their hair blond with dye from the flowers. The Greeks and Romans used saffron to perfume their homes, public buildings, and baths.

- In the 14th through the 18th centuries, saffron was widely used in Europe as a spice and remedy for women's ailments.

- In Chinese medicine, saffron is used to alleviate mental depression and menstrual discomfort.

- The flowers are used as a yellow dye, and the oil is an ingredient in expensive perfumes. Saffron is considered the most expensive spice today. To produce 1 pound of the spice, 35,000–40,000 flowers are required.

Documented Properties

Analgesic, Antineuralgic, Antispasmodic, Aphrodisiac, Diaphoretic, Emmenagogue, Expectorant, Febrifuge, Hepatic, Hypotensor, Nervine, Sedative, Stimulant

Aromatherapy Methods of Use: Fragrancing

CAUTION: Saffron contains toxic components that act on the nervous system; it can also damage the kidneys.

SAGE & SAGE (Spanish)

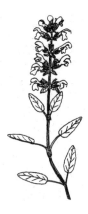

Botanical Name: *Salvia lavandulifolia* (Spanish sage); *Salvia officinalis* (Sage)
Family: *Lamiaceae*

The essential oil is obtained from the flowers and leaves of the plant.

History and Information

- Sage is an evergreen plant native to the Mediterranean region. The plant grows to a height of about 2½ feet, and has aromatic grayish-green leaves and small light-blue to purple flowers. Spanish sage is an evergreen plant native to Spain. It grows to a height of about 2½ feet and has small purple flowers. There are about five hundred different varieties of sage.

- Ancient Egyptian women who were unable to bear children were given sage leaves to help them become pregnant. The herb was also used as a tonic for the brain.

- The Romans called sage *herba sacra*, which means "sacred herb." The Romans and Greeks used sage for snakebites, to invigorate the mind and body, and promote longevity. According to Hippocrates, sage helped women become fertile.

- Sage was included among the herbs Emperor Charlemagne ordered to be grown in his imperial gardens.

- In the Middle Ages, sage was used for constipation, cholera, colds, fever, liver troubles, and epilepsy.

- The Chinese traded three times the amount of their best tea for the Dutch's European sage.

- In the early 1800's, the freshly crushed leaves were used to destroy warts.

- Sage was associated with wisdom, and consumed regularly with the belief that it made one wise and strengthened the memory.

- The American Indians used a salve from the leaves to treat skin sores.

- Many Swiss peasants and Bedouin Arabs rub sage leaves over their teeth to keep them clean and free of yellow film and stains.

- In Europe, sage has been used by women to regulate their menstrual cycle.

- In Latin America, the leaves are rubbed on insect bites to soothe the skin.

- Sage leaves yield 1.5–2.5% essential oil, which is used for its spicy flavor in foods as well as in perfumes and personal-hygiene products.

Practical Uses

Improves circulation
Improves digestion
Purifying; helps in the reduction of cellulite
Reduces stress
Improves alertness
Lessens aches, pains, and menstrual pain, relaxes sore muscles; for general weakness
Suppresses perspiration
Suppresses lactation

Documented Properties

Antibacterial, Antidepressant, Antidiabetic, Antifungal, Antigalactagogue, Anti-inflammatory, Antioxidant, Antirheumatic, Antiseptic, Antispasmodic, Antisudorific, Antiviral, Aperitif, Aperitive, Astringent, Blood Purifier, Carminative, Cholagogue, Cicatrizant, Depurative, Digestive, Disinfectant (*Strong*), Diuretic, Emmenagogue, Estrogenic, Euphoriant, Expectorant, Febrifuge, Healing, Hemostatic (*Bleeding Gums*), Hepatic, Hypertensor, Insect Repellent, Laxative, Nervine, Stimulant (*Brain; Circulatory System; Adrenal Glands*), Stomachic, Tonic (*Digestive System*), Vermifuge, Vulnerary, Warming

Aromatherapy Methods of Use: Application, aroma lamp, bath, diffusor, inhaler, light bulb ring, massage, mist spray

CAUTION: Sage oil contains a toxic component called thujone, which can interfere with brain and nervous system functions. Spanish sage is less toxic and safer to use. Both common sage and Spanish sage should not be used by people prone to epileptic seizures.

SANDALWOOD

Botanical Name: *Santalum album*
Family: *Santalaceae*

The essential oil is obtained from the inner wood of the tree.

History and Information

- Sandalwood is an evergreen tree native to Asia. The tree grows to a height of about 30 feet, and has small purple flowers and small fruits containing a seed. There are ten species of sandalwood trees.

- Sandalwood has been used throughout history in medicine, perfumery, cosmetics, and incense. Since ancient times, sandalwood has been very sacred to the people of India, who used the wood to make furniture, caskets, and canes. Temples were built with the wood because of its fragrant scent and insect-resistant property.

- Today, the Indian government owns all the sandalwood trees grown in India in order to keep them from extinction. Government inspectors allow the extraction of the oil only after the tree has turned 30 years old and grown 30 feet in height.

- The oil is used extensively in Oriental funeral ceremonies and religious rites.

- Sandalwood is used as a fixative in perfumes, soaps, lotions, detergents, and is burned as incense. It is also added to flavor foods, candies, beverages, baked goods, and liqueurs.

- The roots and wood yield about 6% oil, while the leaves and shoots yield about 4% oil.

Practical Uses

Calming, relaxing; reduces stress, promotes a restful sleep
Soothing to the breathing passages
Mood uplifting, aphrodisiac, euphoric; brings out emotions; helps one to dream; helpful for meditation
Used as a fixative to hold the scent of a fragrance
Healing and moisturizing to the skin

Documented Properties

Analgesic, Antibacterial, Antidepressant, Antifungal, Anti-inflammatory, Antiphlogistic, Antipruritic, Antiseptic, Antispasmodic, Antistress, Antiviral, Aphrodisiac, Astringent, Calmative, Carminative, Cicatrizant, Decongestant, Deodorant, Diaphoretic, Diuretic, Emollient, Euphoriant, Expectorant, Febrifuge, Fixative, Healing (*Skin*), Insect Repellent, Relaxant, Sedative, Stimulant, Stomachic, Tonic

Aromatherapy Methods of Use: Application, aroma lamp, bath, inhaler, light bulb ring, massage, mist spray, steam inhalation, steam and sauna room

SANTOLINA (Lavender Cotton)

Botanical Name: *Lavandula taemina, Santolina chamaecyparissus*
Family: *Asteraceae*

The essential oil is obtained from the seeds of the plant.

History and Information

- Santolina is an evergreen plant native to Italy. The plant grows to a height of about 2 feet, and has silver-gray leaves and yellow daisy-like flowers. The entire plant is fragrant. Santolina is a member of the daisy family and is not related to lavender, even though it is referred to as lavender cotton.

- Pliny, the Roman herbalist, recommended santolina for snakebites.

- During medieval times, santolina was used to promote menstruation, purify the kidneys, and for worms and jaundice.

- The plant was used as an air freshener in the Mediterranean area.

Documented Properties

Anthelmintic, Antifungal, Antiphlogistic, Antiseptic, Antispasmodic, Antitoxic, Diuretic, Emmenagogue, Insect Repellent, Hepatic, Parasiticide, Refreshing, Stimulant, Stomachic, Tonic, Vermifuge, Vulnerary

Aromatherapy Methods of Use: Fragrancing

CAUTION: Santolina oil is toxic.

SASSAFRAS

Botanical Name:
Sassafras albidum
Family: *Lauraceae*

The essential oil is obtained from the bark of the tree.

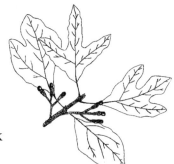

History and Information

- Sassafras is native to North America. The tree grows to a height of about 65–125 feet. Sassafras produces clusters of small yellow flowers, which develop into egg-shaped, dark blue berries. The tree's powerful roots can penetrate rocks.

- The bark was used as a folk remedy for stomachaches, gout, muscle and joint aches, colds, fevers, and to reduce lactation; the oil also helped warm muscles and kill lice.

- In dentistry, the oil was used as an antiseptic. Sassafras has also been used to flavor toothpaste, mouthwashes, root beer, and chewing gum, and scent perfume and soaps.

- The bark contains approximately 7% essential oil.

Practical Uses

Purifying; helps in the reduction of cellulite
Relieves aches, pains, and inflammations; loosens tight muscles
Stimulates the liver

Documented Properties

Alterative, Antidote, Antigalactagogue, Antispasmodic, Blood Purifier, Carminative, Depurative, Diaphoretic, Digestive, Diuretic, Emmenagogue, Febrifuge, Hypotensor, Insect Repellent, Stimulant (*Mild*), Tonic, Warming

CAUTION: Sassafras oil is toxic.

SAVORY

Botanical Name: *Calamintha montana, Satureja montana, S. obovata* (Winter savory); *Calamintha hortensis, Satureja hortensis* (Summer savory)
Family: *Lamiaceae*

The essential oil is obtained from the plant.

History and Information

- Savory is an evergreen tree native to Europe and Asia. The plant grows to a height of about 1 foot, and has small aromatic grayish leaves that turn purple (in late summer) and white, pink, or violet flowers. There are thirty species of savory.

- The Egyptians and Romans used savory as an aphrodisiac in love potions. The Roman men mixed the herb with melted beeswax and made it into a massage lotion to help entice unromantic women. (Hurley, Judith Benn. *The Good Herb.* William Morrow Company, 1995. p. 250)

- During the medieval times, the plants were strewn throughout households to freshen the air.

- Savory was used in medications to treat mouth and throat ulcers.

- Herbalists recommended savory for insect stings and to aid digestion.

- The leaves yield 1% essential oil.

Practical Uses

Warming; improves circulation
Relieves pain

Documented Properties

Analgesic, Antibacterial, Antifungal, Antiputrid, Antiseptic, Antispasmodic, Antiviral, Aperitive, Aphrodisiac, Astringent, Carminative, Cicatrizant, Digestive, Disinfectant, Emmenagogue, Expectorant, Irritant (*Skin*), Parasiticide, Resolvent, Revitalizing, Rubefacient, Stimulant (*Circulatory, Digestive, and Nervous Systems; Adrenal Glands*), Tonic, Vermifuge

Aromatherapy Methods of Use: Application, massage

CAUTION: Savory oil can irritate the skin and should either be avoided or used with extra care by people who have sensitive skin. Use small amounts.

SPEARMINT

Botanical Name: *Mentha spicata, M. viridis*
Family: *Lamiaceae*

The essential oil is obtained from the leaves and flowering tops of the plant.

History and Information

- Spearmint is native to the Mediterranean region. The plant grows to a height of about 1–3 feet, and has shiny green leaves and white or lilac flowers.

- Spearmint has been used for centuries by Egyptian, Greek, and Roman physicians. The

Romans wore mint wreaths in their hair during banquets and decorated their tables with the twigs.

- Hippocrates mentioned mint for its diuretic and stimulant properties.

- Pliny, the Roman herbalist, mentioned spearmint in forty-one different potions. Specifically, he recommended its use as a restorative to vitalize the body and aid digestion.

- Spearmint leaves were strewn on the streets by the Romans to congratulate triumphant gladiators.

- Galen, the Greek physician, considered mint to be an aphrodisiac.

- During the Middle Ages, powdered mint leaves were used to whiten teeth, heal animal and insect bites, prevent milk from curdling, heal mouth sores, and repel mice and rats.

- The American Indians used the leaves to aid digestion, relieve headaches, fevers, sore throats, and diarrhea.

- Spearmint is renowned for its use to help overcome frigidity in both males and females. It is given to bulls and stallions to encourage sexual interest.

Practical Uses

Cooling
Improves digestion; increases appetite; relieves flatulence, freshens the breath and the intestines
Stimulates and strengthens the nerves
Vapors open sinus and breathing passages
Mood uplifting, refreshing, reviving, aphrodisiac; stimulates the metabolism, increases physical strength and endurance; improves mental clarity, alertness, and the memory, sharpens the senses; encourages communication
Relieves aches, pains, inflammation, and menstrual pain
Repels insects
Soothes itching skin

Documented Properties

Analgesic, Antidepressant, Antigalactagogue, Antipruritic, Antiseptic, Antispasmodic, Antitoxic, Aperitive, Aphrodisiac, Astringent, Carminative, Cephalic, Cholagogue, Decongestant, Diaphoretic, Digestive, Diuretic, Emmenagogue, Expectorant, Febrifuge, Hepatic, Insecticide, Nervine, Refreshing, Refrigerant, Restorative, Reviving, Stimulant (*Nervous and Digestive Systems*), Stomachic, Tonic

Aromatherapy Methods of Use: Application, aroma lamp, diffusor, inhaler, light bulb ring, massage, mist spray, steam inhalation, steam and sauna room

CAUTION: Spearmint oil can irritate the skin and should either be avoided or used with extra care by people who have sensitive skin. Use small amounts. Avoid using before bedtime since the oil can overstimulate the nervous system.

SPIKENARD

Botanical Name: *Nardostachys jatamansi*
Family: *Valerianaceae*

The essential oil is obtained from the roots of the plant.

History and Information

- Spikenard is native to the Himalaya Mountains and Asia. The aromatic plant grows to a height of about 2 feet and has pink bell-shaped flowers. Spikenard is also known as musk root.

- The herb was highly prized by the Romans as a perfume.

- In Ayurvedic medicine, spikenard is said to facilitate birth and darken the hair.

- Spikenard oil is also referred to as nard oil. The properties of the oil are similar to valerian.

Practical Uses

Calming, relaxing, reduces stress; promotes a restful sleep

Mood uplifting
Reduces inflammation

Documented Properties

Analgesic, Antibacterial, Antifungal, Anti-inflammatory, Antiseptic, Antispasmodic, Aperitif, Calmative, Carminative, Diuretic, Emmenagogue, Laxative, Sedative, Tonic, Tranquilizer

Aromatherapy Methods of Use: Application, bath, inhaler, massage, mist spray

SPRUCE, SPRUCE-HEMLOCK & SPRUCE-SITKA

Botanical Name: *Picea mariana* (Spruce); *Tsuga canadensis* (Spruce-hemlock); *Picea sitchensis* (Spruce-sitka)
Family: *Pinaceae*

The essential oil is obtained from the bark and branches of the tree.

History and Information

- Spruce is an evergreen tree native to North America. The tree grows to a height of about 70–200 feet, and has red male and female cones. There are about fifty species in the spruce tree family. It is estimated that the trees can live to an age of 1200 years.

- The American Indians heated the twigs in steam baths to induce sweating for relief of rheumatism, colds, and coughs, and applied the bark and twigs externally to stop bleeding wounds. They also made beer by boiling the spruce twigs and cones in maple syrup. A tea was made from the bark for colds, painful joints, and as a laxative; a poultice was made to reduce inflammations.

- The wood is used for the sounding boards in pianos and for the bodies of violins.

Practical Uses

Calming; reduces stress
Vapors open sinus and breathing passages
Mood uplifting, euphoric; improves mental clari-
ty; brings out inner feelings, encourages communication
Disinfectant

Documented Properties

Anti-inflammatory, Antiseptic, Antispasmodic, Antitussive, Astringent, Diaphoretic, Diuretic, Expectorant, Hemostatic, Nervine, Parasiticide, Rubefacient, Sedative, Tonic, Vulnerary, Warming

Aromatherapy Methods of Use: Application, aroma lamp, bath, diffusor, inhaler, light bulb ring, massage, mist spray, steam inhalation, steam and sauna room

ST. JOHN'S WORT

Botanical Name: *Hypericum perforatum*
Family: *Guttiferae*

The essential oil is obtained from the blossoms of the plant.

History and Information

- St. John's Wort is native to Europe, Asia, and Africa. The plant grows to a height of about 1–3 feet with star-shaped yellow flowers. When the flowers are pinched, the petals turn red.

- The American Indians made a tea from the plant to help respiratory problems.

- In the Middle Ages, St. John's Wort was frequently applied to heal wounds.

- St. John's Wort has been used by herbalists to repair nerve damage and reduce pain and inflammation.

Practical Uses

Soothes the intestines
Calming; reduces stress
Mood uplifting, euphoric; improves mental clarity
Relieves aches, pains, and menstrual discomfort

Documented Properties

Alterative, Analgesic, Antibacterial, Antidepressant, Anti-inflammatory, Antiseptic, Antispasmodic (*Menstrual Cramps*), Antiviral, Astringent,

Blood Purifier, Calmative, Carminative, Diuretic, Emmenagogue, Euphoric, Expectorant, Nervine, Sedative, Stomachic, Tonic (*Nervous System*), Tranquilizer, Vermifuge, Vulnerary

Aromatherapy Methods of Use: Application, aroma lamp, bath, diffusor, inhaler, light bulb ring, massage, mist spray

CAUTION: St. John's Wort is phototoxic. Avoid exposure to direct sunlight several hours after applying the oil on the skin.

STYRAX (Liquidamber or Storax)

Botanical Name: *Balsam styracis, Liquidamber orientalis, L. styraciflua*
Family: *Hamamelidaceae*

The resin/essential oil is obtained from the tree.

History and Information

- Styrax is native to America. The tree grows to a height of about 125–150 feet, and has five pointed star-shaped leaves and small yellow-green flowers that develop into a brown fruit. The styrax resin is secreted under the bark, and is referred to as storax. The tree is also known as sweet gum, red gum, and alligator tree.

- Styrax gum is also derived from the *Liquidamber orientalis* tree, which is native to Asia. The tree grows to a height of up to 40 feet, thrives in warm, hilly locations, and has clusters of yellow flowers that develop into a fruit. The gum is also known as Turkish sweet gum.

- The American pioneers made an ointment from the balsam to relieve hemorrhoids, ringworm, and scalp and skin infections. The bark and leaves were used for diarrhea.

- The American Indians made a preparation of styrax to relieve fevers, inflammations, heal wounds, and for skin itch.

- Guatemala and Honduras are the main suppliers of styrax. It is used to flavor soft drinks, tobacco, candy, chewing gum, to scent perfumes, and as an incense. The tree is grown for its timber for furniture making.

Practical Uses

Helps break down cellulite; removes lymphatic deposits
Calming
Mood uplifting
Reduces inflammation

Documented Properties

Antibacterial, Anti-inflammatory, Antiseptic, Antispasmodic, Antitussive, Astringent, Balsamic, Diuretic, Expectorant, Nervine, Stimulant

Aromatherapy Methods of Use: Application, massage

TAGETES

Botanical Name: *Tagetes erecta, T. minuta, T. patula*
Family: *Asteraceae*

The essential oil is obtained from the plant.

History and Information

- Tagetes is native to America. The plant grows to a height of about 1 foot and produces many flowers. The colors of the flowers on the different varieties of tagetes are yellow, orange, and reddish brown. The plant is also known as French marigold and African marigold.

- The Aztecs used the flowers to lower blood pressure, reduce inflammation, and calm nerves.

- In China, the plant is used for coughs, colds, sores, and ulcers.

- Tagetes is added to chicken feed to give a yellow coloring to the skin of the chicken and the egg yolk.

- The oil is used in perfumery, cosmetics, and for food flavorings.

Practical Uses

Disinfectant
Healing to the skin

Documented Properties

Anthelmintic, Antibacterial, Anti-inflammatory, Antifungal, Antiphlogistic, Antiseptic, Antispasmodic, Carminative, Cytophylactic, Decongestant, Diaphoretic, Dilator, Emmenagogue, Emollient, Hypotensor, Insect Repellent, Insecticide, Parasiticide, Sedative, Stomachic, Tranquilizer

Aromatherapy Methods of Use: Application, aroma lamp, light bulb ring, massage, mist spray

CAUTION: Tagetes oil can irritate the skin and should either be avoided or used with extra care by people who have sensitive skin. Use small amounts. Tagetes is phototoxic. Avoid exposure to direct sunlight several hours after applying the oil on the skin.

TARRAGON (Estragon)

Botanical Name: *Artemisia dracunculus*
Family: *Asteraceae*

The essential oil is obtained from the plant.

History and Information

- Tarragon is native to Russia. The shrubby plant grows to a height of about 2–3 feet and has light-green flowers.

- Pliny, the Roman herbalist, claimed the herb prevented fatigue.

- In the Middle Ages, sprigs of tarragon were placed in the shoes before beginning long trips on foot in order to prevent tired feet.

- During the 13th century, tarragon was used by herbalists to sweeten the breath and promote sleep.

- The American Indians made a tea from the plant for diarrhea, colds, headaches, and difficult childbirths.

- The roots of the plant resemble a serpent and were, therefore, used as a treatment for snakebites.

- The plant yields 0.5–1% essential oil. Tarragon is used in perfumes, soaps, cosmetics, and to flavor foods and liqueurs.

Practical Uses

Improves mental clarity and alertness
Relieves aches, pains, and menstrual pain

Documented Properties

Analgesic, Antifungal, Anthelmintic, Anti-inflammatory, Antioxidant, Antirheumatic, Antiseptic, Antispasmodic, Antiviral, Aperitive, Carminative, Cholagogue, Digestive, Diuretic, Emmenagogue, Hepatic, Hypnotic, Laxative, Parasiticide, Stimulant (*Circulatory System*), Stomachic, Tonic, Vermifuge

Aromatherapy Methods of Use: Application, aroma lamp, bath, diffusor, inhaler, light bulb ring, massage, mist spray

CAUTION: Due to the toxicity of the oil, use small amounts.

TEA TREE

Botanical Name: *Melaleuca alternifolia, M. linariifolia, M. uncinata*
Family: *Myrtaceae*

The essential oil is obtained from the leaves and twigs of the tree.

History and Information

- Tea tree is an evergreen tree native to Australia. The tree grows to a height of about 10 feet, and has needle-like leaves and purple or yellow flowers. Tea tree belongs to a family of over 150 species of evergreen trees.

- Tea tree was discovered during the expedition of Captain Cook in 1770. The crew members brewed a tea from the leaves that they enjoyed drinking.

Practical Uses

Vapors open sinus and breathing passages
Mood uplifting; reviving; improves mental clarity
Relieves pain
Disinfectant
Healing to the skin; soothes insect bites

Documented Properties

Analgesic, Antibacterial, Antifungal, Anti-inflammatory, Antipruritic, Antiseptic (*Strong*), Antiviral, Balsamic, Cicatrizant, Cordial, Decongestant, Diaphoretic, Expectorant, Insecticide, Parasiticide, Refreshing, Revitalizing, Stimulant, Sudorific, Vulnerary

Aromatherapy Methods of Use: Application, aroma lamp, bath, diffusor, inhaler, light bulb ring, massage, mist spray, steam inhalation, steam and sauna room

TEREBINTH

Botanical Name: *Pinus maritima, P. palustris, Pistacia terebinthus,* and other *Pinus* species
Family: *Anacardiaceae (Pistacia species)* and *Pinaceae (Pinus species)*

The essential oil is obtained from the sap of the tree bark.

History and Information

- Terebinth is native to the Mediterranean region. The resin is extracted from a large variety of trees, including *Pistacia terebinthus* and various pine trees.

- The people of the Near East chewed terebinth to strengthen their teeth and gums.

Practical Uses

Vapors open sinus and breathing passages
Refreshing, reviving; improves mental clarity
Lessens aches and pains
Disinfectant
Repels insects

Documented Properties

Analgesic, Antidote, Antipruritic, Antirheumatic, Antiseptic, Antispasmodic, Balsamic, Carminative, Cicatrizant, Counter-irritant, Diuretic, Expectorant, Healing, Hemostatic, Insecticide, Laxative, Parasiticide, Rubefacient, Stimulant, Tonic, Vermifuge

Aromatherapy Methods of Use: Application, aroma lamp, bath, diffusor, inhaler, light bulb ring, massage, mist spray, steam inhalation, steam and sauna room

THUJA (Cedar Leaf)

Botanical Name: *Thuja occidentalis*
Family: *Cupressaceae*

The essential oil is obtained from the leaves, bark, and twigs of the tree.

History and Information

- Thuja is an evergreen tree native to China and North America. The tree grows to a height of about 65 feet. Thuja is also known as arbor vitae or northern white cedar.

- The Egyptians made coffins from the wood and used the oil for embalming.

- The North American Indians used thuja to remedy menstrual discomforts, headaches, and heart problems. The twigs were also made into a tea for rheumatism.

Documented Properties

Anthelmintic, Antirheumatic, Antiseptic, Antiviral, Astringent, Cicatrizant, Counter-irritant, Diuretic, Emmenagogue, Expectorant, Hemostatic, Hypotensor, Insect Repellent, Parasiticide (*Skin*), Rubefacient, Stimulant (*Nerves*), Sudorific, Tonic, Vermifuge

COMMENTS: The oil is approved for use in food provided its toxic component, thujone, is removed.

CAUTION: Thuja oil is toxic due to the high content of thujone, which can interfere with brain and nervous system functions.

THYME

Botanical Name: *Thymus aestivus, T. citriodora, T. ilerdensis, T. satureiodes, T. valentianus, T. vulgaris, T. vulgaris* var. *linalol, T. webbianus*
Family: *Lamiaceae*

The essential oil is obtained from the leaves and flowering tops of the plant.

History and Information

- Thyme is an evergreen plant native to the Mediterranean region. The plant grows to a height of about 1 foot, and has small leaves and pink or pale lilac flowers.

- The thymus gland was named after the Latin name *thymus* because the gland's appearance resembled the thyme flower.

- Since ancient times, thyme has been used in Egypt, Greece, and Rome. The Greeks used thyme for nervous conditions and to invigorate the senses. Thyme was burned to repel insects and used to preserve meats. The Roman soldiers would bathe in water with thyme added to gain vigor and courage. Thyme was associated with courage well into the Middle Ages.

- Herbalists of the Middle Ages recommended thyme for melancholy, epilepsy, nightmares, to help urination problems, strengthen the lungs, improve digestion, and for female problems.

- From the 15th to the 17th century, when the plague devastated the people of Europe, thyme was used as a germicide. Members of the nobility carried posies of aromatic herbs, including thyme, to protect themselves from the germs of the public.

- In World War I, thymol, derived from thyme, was used as an antiseptic to treat the wounds of the soldiers. In addition, thymol was used to purify the air in hospitals and sickrooms.

- Bees are attracted to thyme, and the honey they produce has been a longtime favorite in Europe.

- In Germany today, thyme preparations are used to clear chest congestion.

- The herb yields approximately 1% essential oil. The oil is extensively used in perfumery, cosmetics, liqueurs, and to flavor foods.

Practical Uses

Heating; increases circulation
Improves digestion; cleanses the intestines
Purifying; removes cellulite, waste material and excessive fluids from the body
Relaxes the nerves
Vapors open the sinus and breathing passages
Mood uplifting; improves mental clarity and alertness, sharpens the senses
Stimulates the thyroid gland; increases physical endurance and energy
Relieves aches, pains, inflammation, and spasms
Induces perspiration
Disinfectant
Repels insects and kills lice

Documented Properties

Analgesic, Anthelmintic, Antibacterial, Antidepressant, Anti-inflammatory, Antifungal, Antioxidant, Antipruritic, Antiputrid, Antirheumatic, Antiseptic (*Strong*), Antispasmodic, Antitoxic, Antitussive, Antivenomous, Antiviral, Aperitif, Aphrodisiac, Astringent, Balsamic, Bronchodilator, Cardiac, Carminative, Cicatrizant, Counterirritant, Cytophylactic, Diaphoretic, Digestive, Diuretic, Emmenagogue, Expectorant, Hypertensor, Insecticide, Nervine, Parasiticide, Pectoral, Rubefacient, Sedative, Stimulant, Stomachic, Sudorific, Tonic, Uplifting, Vermifuge, Warming

Aromatherapy Methods of Use: Application, aroma lamp, bath (only the *linalol* variety), diffusor, inhaler, light bulb ring, massage, mist spray, steam inhalation

COMMENTS: The varieties of lemon-scented thyme (*Thymus citriodora*), *Thymus satureiodes,* and *Thymus linalol (Thymus vulgaris* var. *linalol)* are less irritating to the skin and less toxic than common thyme.

CAUTION: Thyme oil can irritate the skin and should either be avoided or used with extra care by people who have sensitive skin. Use small amounts. Thyme should not be used by people prone to epileptic seizures.

TOBACCO LEAF

Botanical Name: *Nicotiana tabacum*
Family: *Solanaceae*

The CO_2 extract is obtained from the leaves of the plant.

History and Information

- Tobacco is a flowering perennial plant native to the Americas and West Indies. the plant thrives in rich, moist soil and reaches a height of about 3–15 feet. Depending on the variety, the flowers are pink, green, or white, and emit their fragrant scent after dark. There are nearly one hundred species of *Nicotiana*.

- The American Indians were the first to grow and smoke tobacco. They believed that tobacco possessed medicinal properties and burned the leaves as incense during their ceremonies.

- The genus *Nicotiana* was named in honor of Jean Nicot, a French ambassador to Portugal, who played a significant role in influencing the spread of tobacco use in Europe.

Practical Uses

Calms hysteria
Dulls the senses
Aphrodisiac

Aromatherapy Methods of Use: Application

CAUTION: Tobacco leaf oil is toxic.

TOLU BALSAM

Botanical Name: *Myroxlon balsamum*
Family: *Fabaceae*

The resin/essential oil is obtained from the bark of the tree.

History and Information

- Tolu is an evergreen tree native to Central and South America. The tree grows to a maximum height of about 120 feet and has small white flowers that develop into fruits. The resin is obtained by making an incision in the tree.

- The use of tolu balsam dates back to the 1500's when it was added to cough medicines for its expectorant effect.

- Tolu balsam is used to flavor foods and soft drinks, and to fragrance perfumes and soaps. Some of the trees are grown for timber. The wood, resembling mahogany, is hard and strong, and used for making furniture.

Practical Uses

Mood uplifting
Used as a fixative to hold the scent of a fragrance; also as a deodorant

Documented Properties

Antiseptic, Expectorant, Fixative

Aromatherapy Methods of Use: Application, massage, mist spray

TONKA BEAN (Tonquin Bean)

Botanical Name: *Baryosma tongo, Coumarouna odorata, Dipteryx odorata*
Family: *Fabaceae*

The essential oil is obtained from the beans of the tree.

History and Information

- Tonka is native to South America. The tree grows to a height of about 100 feet and has red fragrant flowers that develop into fruits, which contain a few strongly-fragrant black seeds called tonka beans. During the drying process, the fragrance of the beans intensifies. The bark and the wood are odorless.

- Tonka bean is used for flavoring foods and as a vanilla substitute in perfumery. In Europe, an insecticide product is made from the beans.

Practical Uses

Calming
Mood uplifting

Documented Properties

Insecticide

Aromatherapy Methods of Use: Application, aroma lamp, fragrancing, light bulb ring, inhaler, massage, mist spray

CAUTION: Tonka bean oil is toxic.

TUBEROSE

Botanical Name: *Polianthes tuberosa*
Family: *Agavaceae*

The absolute/essential oil is obtained from the flowers of the plant.

History and Information

- Tuberose is native to Asia and Central America. The plant produces strongly-fragrant white flowers that bloom in the summer. There are thirteen species of tuberose that belong to the agave family.

- Tuberose has long been a symbol of seductiveness. Early writers warned young girls to avoid smelling the fragrance of the flowers because the scent would make them vulnerable. The Malays called the fragrance "Mistress of the Night" because its scent intensifies after sunset.

Documented Properties

Nervine, Uplifting

Aromatherapy Methods of Use: Application, fragrancing, massage

TURMERIC

Botanical Name: *Amomoum curcuma, Curcuma domestica, C. longa*
Family: *Zingiberaceae*

The essential oil is obtained from the plant root.

History and Information

- Turmeric is native to Asia. The plant grows to a height of about 3 feet and has yellow flowers. The root is bright orange with a thin brownish skin. The rhizomes provide the spice. Turmeric belongs to the same family as ginger.

- Turmeric has been used as a spice and dye since biblical times.

- The plant was called Indian saffron during the Middle Ages because of its orange-yellow color.

- In Chinese and Ayurvedic medicine, turmeric root has been used to stimulate circulation, improve digestion, ease menstrual problems, and relieve aches, pains, and inflammation.

- Turmeric is used in Oriental-type perfumes and to flavor food products; it is an ingredient in curry powder and various mustards.

Practical Uses

Warming; increases circulation
Calming, relaxing; reduces stress, promotes a restful sleep
Mood uplifting; improves mental clarity

Documented Properties

Analgesic, Anthelmintic, Antiarthritic, Antibacterial, Anti-inflammatory, Antioxidant (*Strong*), Aphrodisiac, Carminative, Cholagogue, Digestive, Diuretic, Hepatic, Hypotensive, Insecticidal, Laxative, Rubefacient, Stimulant

Aromatherapy Methods of Use: Application, aroma lamp, diffusor, light bulb ring, massage, mist spray

CAUTION: Turmeric oil is moderately toxic; use in small amounts.

VALERIAN

Botanical Name: *Valeriana officinalis*
Family: *Valerianaceae*

The essential oil is obtained from the plant roots.

History and Information

- Valerian is native to Europe and Asia. The plant grows to a height of about 4–5 feet, and has clusters of small pink or white flowers. Valerian is also known as "all-heal."

- Since ancient times, valerian has been used as a medicinal herb in the treatment of epilepsy, and as a calmative for nervous disorders and hysteria.

- American Indian warriors used valerian as an antiseptic for wounds.

- The oil is used in cosmetics, perfumery, and as a food flavoring. The herb is a leading over-the-counter tranquilizer in Europe.

Practical Uses

Calming; promotes a restful sleep
Relieves pain

Documented Properties

Analgesic, Antibacterial, Anticonvulsive, Antidepressant, Antidiuretic, Antipyretic, Antispasmodic, Carminative, Diuretic, Febrifuge, Hepatic, Hypotensor, Nervine, Sedative (*Strong*), Stomachic, Tonic (*Strong*) (*Nerves*), Tranquilizer, Vermifuge

Aromatherapy Methods of Use: Application, aroma lamp, inhaler, massage, mist spray

VANILLA

Botanical Name: *Vanilla fragrans, V. planifolia*
Family: *Orchidaceae*

The absolute/essential oil is obtained from the unripe pods of the plant.

History and Information

- Vanilla is native to Mexico and Central America. The climbing plant reaches a height of about 12 feet and has clusters of flowers.

- The Spaniards, learning that the Aztecs of Mexico used vanilla to flavor cocoa, introduced its use into Europe.

- European physicians used vanilla during the 16th and 17th centuries as an antidote for poisoning, stomach complaints, and as an aphrodisiac.

- Vanilla is used in pharmaceutical products, cosmetics, and foods.

Practical Uses

Calming; reduces stress; promotes a restful sleep
Mood uplifting, aphrodisiac; helps one to dream

Documented Properties

Aphrodisiac, Balsamic, Calmative, Emmenagogue

Aromatherapy Methods of Use: Application, aroma lamp, bath, inhaler, light bulb ring, massage, mist spray

VETIVER

Botanical Name: *Andropogon muricatus, Vetiveria zizanoides*
Family: *Poaceae*

The essential oil is obtained from the roots of the grass.

History and Information

- Vetiver is native to Asia. The tropical grass grows to a height of about 4–8 feet. Since the strong roots reach deep below the soil, it is often planted to protect steep hillsides and other areas vulnerable to soil erosion.

- In India, the plant is known as khas. It is hung over windows and placed into clothing to repel insects. Vetiver is also used as a food flavoring.

- In Russia, the oil is placed in sachets and sewn into the linings of fur coats to protect against damage caused by moths.

- Vetiver oil is used extensively as a fixative in perfumery.

- The roots yield a small amount of oil; therefore, it is often adulterated with synthetics. In the 1970's, vetiver oil was restricted in many countries because of problems with adulteration.

Practical Uses

Improves digestion
Calms nervousness, relieves stress and tension; promotes a restful sleep
Mood uplifting
Strengthens the body
Relieves pain, loosens tight muscles
Repels insects
Used as a fixative to hold the scent of a fragrance
Healing to the skin

Documented Properties

Antiseptic, Antispasmodic, Antistress, Aphrodisiac, Calmative, Detoxifier, Emmenagogue, Insect Repellent, Nervine, Parasiticide, Revitalizing, Rubefacient, Sedative, Stimulant (*Immune System*), Tonic, Vermifuge

Aromatherapy Methods of Use: Application, aroma lamp, bath, inhaler, light bulb ring, massage, mist spray

VIOLET

Botanical Name: *Viola odorata*
Family: *Violaceae*

The oleoresin/essential oil is obtained from the flowers of the plant.

History and Information

- Violet is native to Europe and Africa. The plant grows to a height of about 6 inches, and has heart-shaped leaves and sweetly-fragrant dark-violet flowers.

- Pliny, the Roman herbalist, recommended violets to relieve headaches, and to calm and induce sleep.

- The Romans and Greeks enjoyed a wine made from violets.

- Roman women added violets to goat's milk and applied the mixture on their face to beautify their complexion.

- The Greeks regarded violet as the flower of fertility and frequently added it to love potions.

- In the 19th century, fragrances made with violets were the most popular in France and England.

- The aroma of violets can cause a temporary loss of smell.

- The flowers can be cooked or eaten raw in salads. In Europe, the flowers are candied and used in confectionery to decorate desserts.

Practical Uses

Calming; promotes a restful sleep
Mood uplifting

Documented Properties

Analgesic, Antiseptic, Anti-inflammatory, Antirheumatic, Aphrodisiac, Calmative, Diaphoretic, Diuretic, Emetic, Expectorant, Febrifuge, Hypnotic, Laxative, Liver Deconges-

tant, Pectoral, Sedative, Stimulant (*Circulatory System*), Uplifting, Vulnerary

Aromatherapy Methods of Use: Application, aroma lamps, bath, fragrancing, inhaler, light bulb ring, massage, mist spray

WINTERGREEN

Botanical Name: *Gaultheria procumbens*
Family: *Ericaceae*

The essential oil is obtained from the leaves of the plant.

History and Information

- Wintergreen is native to North America. The plant grows to a height of about 6 inches, and has leathery leaves and small white flowers.

- American Indians chewed the leaves to improve breathing.

- Early Americans chewed the roots to prevent tooth decay and used the berries as a tonic.

- Wintergreen contains high amounts of methyl salicylate, which is similar to salicylic acid in aspirin. Wintergreen yields approximately 0.5% essential oil; it is used in toothpaste, chewing gum, root beer, and other soft drinks.

Documented Properties

Analgesic, Anti-inflammatory, Antirheumatic, Antispasmodic, Antitussive, Astringent, Carminative, Diuretic, Emmenagogue, Galactagogue, Stimulant

COMMENTS: Wintergreen oil is often falsified with the synthetic chemical, methyl salicylate.

CAUTION: Wintergreen oil is toxic and can irritate the skin.

WORMWOOD

Botanical Name: *Artemisia absinthium*
Family: *Asteraceae*

The essential oil is obtained from the leaves and flowering tops of the plant.

History and Information

- Wormwood is native to Europe. The plant grows to a height of about 1–4 feet, and has grayish-green aromatic leaves and clusters of small yellow flowers.

- In ancient times, the herb was favored by women because it helped to bring on the menstrual cycle.

- Wormwood was the main ingredient in an alcoholic drink known as absinthe, which was found to be toxic.

Documented Properties

Abortifacient, Anthelmintic, Antidote, Anti-inflammatory, Antipruritic, Antiseptic, Antispasmodic, Aperitive, Cardiac, Carminative, Cholagogue, Choleretic, Diaphoretic, Digestive, Disinfectant, Diuretic, Emmenagogue, Febrifuge, Hepatic, Insect Repellent, Stimulant (*Digestive System*), Stomachic, Tonic, Vermifuge

CAUTION: Wormwood oil contains a component called thujone, which interferes with brain and nervous system functions. The oil is toxic and has been known to induce mental impairment.

YARROW

Botanical Name: *Achillea millefolium*
Family: *Asteraceae*

The essential oil is obtained from the flowering plant.

History and Information

- Yarrow is native to Europe and Asia. The plant grows to a height of about 1–3 feet with white, yellow, lilac, or pink flower heads and feathery leaves.

- In ancient China, yarrow was believed to be a sacred plant.

- The American Indians used the root for pain relief, swellings, itching, and insect bites; the leaves were used to induce perspiration in order to reduce fevers, expel worms, clot the blood, and as a diuretic. The entire plant was used to heal burns, bruises, and for earaches.

- Early Americans chewed the leaves to relieve an upset stomach, regulate menstrual flow, and for fever, chills, rashes, and dreaming.

- In Nordic countries, the plant was substituted for hops in the production of beer. In Germany, the seeds were used as a preservative in wine.

- In China, the herb is used for animal and snakebites.

- The plant contains proazulene, which, when distilled, produces the anti-inflammatory substance, azulene. Since the essential oil of yarrow is said to contain more azulene than chamomile, it is often added to chamomile to increase its azulene content.

- Yarrow yields 0.5% essential oil.

Practical Uses

Calming
Vapors open sinus and breathing passages
Improves mental clarity
Lessens inflammation

Documented Properties

Abortifacient, Analgesic, Anthelmintic, Anti-inflammatory, Antiphlogistic, Antiseptic, Antispasmodic, Aperitive, Astringent, Blood Purifier, Carminative, Cholagogue, Cicatrizant, Diaphoretic, Digestive, Diuretic, Emmenagogue, Expectorant, Febrifuge, Healing, Hemostatic, Hepatic, Hypotensor, Insect Repellent, Laxative, Stimulant (*Circulatory System*), Stomachic, Sudorific, Tonic, Vulnerary

Aromatherapy Methods of Use: Application, aroma lamp, bath, inhaler, light bulb ring, massage, mist spray, steam inhalation, steam and sauna room

YLANG-YLANG

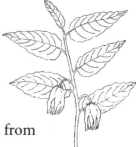

Botanical Name: *Cananga odorata* var. *genuina, Unona odorantissimum*
Family: *Annonaceae*

The essential oil is obtained from the flowers of the tree.

History and Information

- Ylang-Ylang is an evergreen tree native to Asia. The tree grows to a height of about 100 feet, and has glossy leaves and large yellow fragrant flowers.

- The name *ylang-ylang* in the Malayan language means "flower of flowers."

- In Indonesia, ylang-ylang flowers are placed on the bed of a newlywed couple on their wedding night.

- The oil, also known as macassar oil, is a fragrant ingredient in cosmetics, soaps, detergents, lotions, perfumes, beverages, and foods.

Practical Uses

Calming, relaxing, reduces stress; promotes a restful sleep
Mood uplifting, euphoric, aphrodisiac; brings out feelings, enhances communication
Lessens pain, loosens tight muscles
Disinfectant

Documented Properties

Antidepressant, Antipruritic, Antiseptic, Aphrodisiac, Calmative, Carminative, Emmenagogue, Emollient, Euphoriant, Fixative, Hypotensor, Moisturizer, Nervine, Rejuvenator (*Skin and Hair*), Relaxant, Sedative, Stimulant (*Circulatory System*), Tonic

Aromatherapy Methods of Use: Application, aroma lamp, bath, diffusor, fragrancing, inhaler, light bulb ring, massage, mist spray

ZANTHOXYLUM

Botanical Name: *Zanthoxylum alatum, Z. americanum, Z. rhesta*
Family: *Rutaceae*

The essential oil is obtained from the fruit of the tree.

History and Information

- Zanthoxylum is native to Asia and North America. The tree grows to a height of about 10–25 feet and has light-green flowers that develop into small berries. Zanthoxylum belongs to a species of about 250 trees and shrubs, and is in the same family as citrus. The trees are also known as prickly ash.

- The variety *Zanthoxylum americanum* is native to North America. The fruits and bark of the tree were used by the American Indians and early settlers to relieve muscle and joint pains, toothaches, and stomach disorders.

Practical Uses

Warming
Reduces stress and nervous tension; promotes a restful sleep
Vapors open sinus and breathing passages
Mood uplifting, aphrodisiac, euphoric; improves mental clarity
Loosens tight muscles

Documented Properties

Analgesic, Anti-inflammatory, Antiseptic, Diaphoretic, Sedative

Aromatherapy Methods of Use: Application, aroma lamp, bath, inhaler, light bulb ring, massage, mist spray, steam inhalation, sauna and steam room

CHAPTER 4

Infused Oils

Infused oils are made from plant materials that are extracted by the use of heat into a carrier oil medium. Since they are already heavily diluted, these oils can be used without a carrier oil. This method is usually used for plants that yield a very small amount of essential oil.

The following infused oils are covered in this chapter: Aloe Vera, Arnica, Calendula

ALOE VERA

Botanical Name: *Aloe barbadensis, A. vera*
Family: *Liliaceae*

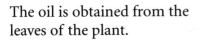

The oil is obtained from the leaves of the plant.

History and Information

- Aloe vera is native to Africa. The plant grows to a height of about 5 feet, and has sword-like leaves and orange-red flowers. There are three hundred varieties of aloe.

- The Arabs were thought to have been the first to master the art of pressing the juice from the plant, which was done with their bare feet.

- Clay tablets in Mesopotamia reveal the use of aloe vera in 1750 B.C.

- The Egyptian Ebers Papyrus from 1550 B.C. described the use of aloe vera for burns, skin ulcers, and infections.

- The Greeks, credited with the early research of aloe in 25 A.D., and were already using it to regulate the bowels.

- In the first century, the Greek physician, Dioscorides, suggested that aloe vera be used to heal skin problems.

- Alexander the Great and Aristotle were known to have enjoyed aloe's soothing and healing effects. It is said that Aristotle asked Alexander the Great to conquer the African island of Socotra in order to obtain a supply of aloe.

- Cleopatra used the gel of the aloe as a cosmetic and skin moisturizer. It is said that aloe vera was one of the main ingredients in her secret beauty cream.

- In Mexican folk medicine, 2 tablespoons of aloe gel are taken to relieve stiff joints.

- In Africa, it is utilized as a purgative for internal systems and to eliminate strong body odors.

- In the United States, aloe is well known for its healing properties of skin tissue.

Practical Uses

Soothing to the digestion
Lessens pain
Healing, moisturizing, and rejuvenating to the skin
Makes the hair more manageable; hydrates dry hair

Documented Properties

Anthelmintic, Antipruritic, Antiseptic, Calmative, Cholagogue, Deodorant, Demulcent, Depurative, Digestive, Emmenagogue, Emollient, Insecticide,

Larvicide, Laxative, Moisturizer, Purgative, Regenerator (*Damaged Tissues*), Stimulant (*Blood Circulation*), Stomachic, Tonic, Vermifuge, Vulnerary

Aromatherapy Methods of Use: Application, massage

COMMENTS: Aloe vera is excellent for healing tissues of any kind.

ARNICA

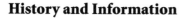

Botanical Name: *Arnica montana*
Family: *Asteraceae*

The infused oil is obtained from the flowers of the plant.

History and Information

- Arnica is native to Europe. The plant grows to a height of about 2 feet and has daisy-like yellow flowers.

- From the early 1800's to 1960, arnica was officially listed in the United States pharmacopoeia for its ability to reduce pain and swelling.

Practical Uses

Lessens pain
Helps injured skin tissue heal faster; wounds and black-and-blue bruises

Documented Properties

Analgesic, Anti-inflammatory, Antispasmodic, Cardiac, Counter-irritant, Diaphoretic, Diuretic, Emollient, Expectorant, Febrifuge, Healing (*Sprains; Dislocations; Fractures*), Hypertensor, Rubefacient, Stimulant (*Circulatory System*), Tonic, Vulnerary

Aromatherapy Methods of Use: Application

CAUTION: Arnica is not recommended to be used on an open cut or wound; use only on unbroken skin. The oil is toxic.

CALENDULA (Marigold)

Botanical Name: *Calendula officinalis*
Family: *Asteraceae*

The infused oil is obtained from the flowers of the plant.

History and Information

- Calendula is native to Central America and Europe. The plant grows to a height of about 3 feet, and has leathery leaves and large yellow-orange or reddish flowers with a strong scent. There are about fifty species of the marigold plant.

- South American Incas planted marigolds together with other plants to reduce insect damage.

- Since the earliest times, calendula has been grown throughout Europe to flavor soups and stews.

- During the Civil War, European settlers came to America and used the plant to stop bleeding and promote the healing of wounds.

- The Arabs feed marigold flowers to their thoroughbred ponies to keep their circulatory vessels healthy. These ponies are highly esteemed all over the world.

Practical Uses

Skin eruptions, eczema, insect bites and stings, bruises, boils, corns, acne, damaged skin and tissue, burns, sunburns; chapped, sensitive, rough, inflamed skin

Documented Properties

Analgesic, Antibacterial, Antifungal, Anti-inflammatory, Antiseptic, Antispasmodic, Aperient, Astringent, Blood Purifier, Cholagogue, Diaphoretic, Digestive, Emmenagogue, Healing, Hepatic, Hemostatic, Stimulant (*Mild*) (*Circulatory System*), Tonic, Tonifying (*Skin*), Vermifuge, Vulnerary

Aromatherapy Methods of Use: Application, massage

CHAPTER 5

Methods of: Application, Dispersion, and Inhalation of Essential Oils

APPLICATION

The self-application method is used when there is not another person available to give a massage, or when a massage is not necessary. The oils should be rubbed into the skin until they are fully absorbed. Then a small amount of cornstarch can be applied over the area so that the skin does not remain greasy.

AROMA LAMP

An aroma lamp has a small container that is heated after water and essential oils are added. When the water becomes hot, the aromatic vapors are dispersed into the air.

BATHS

The combination of a warm bath with essential oils can serve as a delightful therapeutic measure to either relax and calm, or invigorate and refresh the body. An aromatherapy bath can be so pleasurable that it can become an anticipated and planned-for event.

Instructions: Close the bathroom door and window to keep the essential oil vapors from escaping out of the room. Play soft music that you enjoy listening to. Fill the bathtub with water as warm as you like. Mix the essential oils with the carrier oil. Add the blend to the water when the tub is full. Swirl the water to distribute the oils evenly throughout the tub and enter the bath immediately.

DIFFUSORS

Diffusors disperse a mist of microparticles of essential oil, which creates an aromatic atmos-
phere for the indoors. There are different types of diffusors on the market. You can choose a smaller or larger unit, depending on the size of the area to be fragranced. The formulas given for diffusor use in Chapter 6 are in percentages rather than drops because of the different types of units. In one type, essential oils are added to a pad that is vaporized by an electric fan. Another type has a small glass bottle that essential oils are placed into. The oil is then propelled into a nebulizer and vaporized into the air.

INHALERS

This method is handy for quick results.

Instructions: Mix the essential oils in a small glass bottle and tighten the cap.

To use: Open the bottle and slowly inhale the vapors fifteen to twenty times. Cap the bottle immediately after use.

LIGHT BULB RING

A light bulb ring is placed on the top of a cool light bulb and the essential oils are placed into the groove. When the light is turned on, the heated bulb disperses the aromatic vapors into the air.

MASSAGE

An aromatherapy massage can provide a means of counteracting pressures of daily life. Only after receiving a massage do we realize how tight our muscles have been and the high amounts of tension stored in our body. Some people think of massage as a luxury and utilize it only when in severe distress. But living under the strain of modern society, we should recognize massage as an extraordinarily beneficial measure for stressed individuals to receive on a regular basis.

For best results when giving or receiving a massage, please follow these guidelines:

- The room should be quiet, warm, and comfortable.

- Soft music can be played to promote relaxation.

- Mist a nice essential oil fragrance in the room before the treatment.

- Make sure to be in a calm state before giving the massage. Tension can be easily transferred from one person to another.

- Fingernails should be short to avoid scratching the skin.

- A firm cushion can be used if a massage table is unavailable. The recipient should be covered with a sheet or blanket for warmth.

- Choose the appropriate aromatherapy massage formula and place all oils nearby to avoid searching for them during the treatment.

- Wash hands with warm/hot water before and after giving the massage.

- Wear comfortable clothing.

- Warm the carrier/base oil by placing the small container in warm water. Pour an ample amount into the palms of your hands, rub them together, and then apply the oil on the person's skin.

MIST SPRAYS

A convenient and effective way to disperse aromatic vapors in the air is through the use of a mist spray. As the aromas mature in the bottle, the fragrance improves and becomes stronger.

Instructions: Fill a 4-ounce fine mist spray bottle with purified water and add the essential oils. Tighten the cap and shake well.

To use: Shake the bottle well. Sit comfortably in a chair. Close your eyes and begin to take slow deep breaths as you spray the mist approximately ten times over your head (two to three sprays at a time).

SKIN AND HAIR CARE

Many excellent and efficacious skin and hair care products can be easily made with unrefined carrier/base oils, vegetable butters, pure essential oils, and resins.

STEAM INHALATION

This method is usually employed to open the breathing passages.

Instructions: Heat a small pot of water and pour into a bowl, then add the essential oils. Immediately drape a towel over your head, close your eyes, and lean over towards the vapors. Inhale deeply.

STEAM AND SAUNA ROOM

You can transform a sweaty-smelling steam or sauna room into a delightfully uplifting and refreshing atmosphere.

Instructions for a steam room with rocks as a heat source: Add the essential oil blend to a container of water and toss it over the hot rocks. Please be careful not to be splashed as the water hits the rocks.

Instructions for other steam and sauna rooms: Spray the mist away from your body and face to ensure that it does not come in direct contact with your skin or eyes, since the oils can become very irritating to the skin, especially in the hot steam and sauna room.

CHAPTER 6

Making Your Own Aromatic Blends

Across the world, more people are discovering the value of the essential oils. From relative obscurity in the 1980's, aromatherapy has rapidly become more widely recognized and respected by people all over for its effectiveness. Small shops and boutiques are springing up everywhere selling aromatherapy oils and products. Large department stores now proudly proclaim to carry products made with pure essential oils. It is so heartening to be part of the changing trend in which people are returning to a closer connection with nature.

Aromatherapy offers a wonderful opportunity for us to prepare our own blends with pure, natural oils that are beneficial to our health and well-being. There are many ways to capture the benefits of the essential oils. They can be blended for use in a body massage, baths, air fragrancing, inhalers, room disinfectants, skin and hair care, and so much more. These natural oils are extremely versatile and their uses can stretch as far as our imagination. Every day presents us with new opportunities to enjoy the benefits derived from these precious substances; the extent to which we take advantage of them to enhance our lives is completely up to us.

Formulas in this chapter are:

Aches and Pains	Hair Care	Skin Care Creme
Air Fragrancing	Mental Clarity	Sleep Restfully
Breathe Easy	Mood Uplifting	Steam and Sauna Room
Calming	Muscle, Release Tightness	Stress-Free
Car Alert	Nail Conditioner	Warming
Dreams	Romance	
Facial Creme	Room Disinfectant	

Before blending and using any of these formulas, please carefully read Chapter 1 on the safe use of oils. For mixing instructions, please refer to Chapter 5.

ACHES AND PAINS

MASSAGE

Massage into the specific area(s) until the oil is fully absorbed into the skin.

Cabreuva	5 drops	Peppermint	5 drops
Litsea Cubeba	5 drops	Rosemary	4 drops
Palmarosa	5 drops	Geranium	4 drops
Eucalyptus	5 drops	Gingergrass	4 drops
Carrier Oil	4 teaspoons	Cedarwood (*Atlas*)	3 drops
		Carrier Oil	4 teaspoons

♦   ♦   ♦

Cananga	5 drops
Palmarosa	4 drops
Marjoram	4 drops
St. John's Wort	4 drops
Lavender	3 drops
Carrier Oil	4 teaspoons

♦   ♦   ♦

Ravensara Anisata	5 drops
Spearmint	5 drops
Gingergrass	5 drops
Cabreuva	3 drops
Pepper (*Black*)	2 drops
Carrier Oil	4 teaspoons

AIR FRAGRANCING

AROMA LAMPS

Pour water into the container and heat, then drop in the essential oils.

Litsea Cubeba	10 drops
Clove (*Bud*)	5 drops
Cedarwood (*Atlas*)	5 drops

♦   ♦   ♦

Spearmint	10 drops
Cassia	5 drops
Cedarwood (*Atlas*)	5 drops

♦   ♦   ♦

Cassia	5 drops
Orange	5 drops
Amyris	5 drops
Clove (*Bud*)	5 drops

♦   ♦   ♦

Spearmint	7 drops
Cinnamon Bark	5 drops
Clove (*Bud*)	5 drops
Cajeput	3 drops

♦   ♦   ♦

Lemongrass	10 drops
Patchouli	10 drops

♦   ♦   ♦

Spruce	7 drops
Rosemary	7 drops
Cedarwood (*Atlas*)	6 drops

DIFFUSOR

Place the oils in the glass bottle or on the pad, depending on the type of diffusor you have.

Tangerine	50%
Citronella	30%
Clove (*Bud*)	20%

♦   ♦   ♦

Grapefruit	40%
Bergamot	40%
Temple Orange	20%

♦   ♦   ♦

Spearmint	40%
Palmarosa	30%
Clove (*Bud*)	30%

♦   ♦   ♦

Spearmint	40%
Fennel	30%
Allspice	30%

LIGHT BULB RINGS

Place the light bulb ring on a cool light bulb and drop the oils carefully into the grove. Turn the light on and enjoy the aroma.

Spearmint	5 drops
Cassia	5 drops

♦   ♦   ♦

Orange	5 drops
Lime	3 drops
Patchouli	2 drops

✦ ✦ ✦

Orange	7 drops
Juniper Berries	3 drops
Frankincense	3 drops

✦ ✦ ✦

Elemi	5 drops
Clove	3 drops
Spruce	2 drops

✦ ✦ ✦

Spearmint	5 drops
Elemi	5 drops

✦ ✦ ✦

Ylang-Ylang	5 drops
Sandalwood	3 drops
Tangerine	2 drops

MIST SPRAYS

Fill a fine mist spray bottle with purified water and then add the essential oils. Tighten the cap, shake well, and mist numerous times in the air.

Citronella	35 drops
Patchouli	30 drops
Tangerine	30 drops
Bois de Rose	30 drops
Pure Water	4 ounces

✦ ✦ ✦

Lime	50 drops
Spearmint	50 drops
Cedarwood (*Atlas*)	25 drops
Pure Water	4 ounces

✦ ✦ ✦

Spruce	40 drops
Allspice	40 drops
Rosemary	25 drops
Sandalwood	20 drops
Pure Water	4 ounces

✦ ✦ ✦

Bergamot	40 drops
Bois de Rose	30 drops
Geranium	30 drops
Clove (*Bud*)	25 drops
Pure Water	4 ounces

BREATHE EASY

BATHS

Fill the bathtub with water as warm as you like. Mix the formula together, pour into the bathwater, and disperse the oil so that it is distributed evenly. Enjoy your bath for 30 minutes.

Cajeput	4 drops
Tangerine	3 drops
Eucalyptus	3 drops
Leptospermum	2 drops
Carrier Oil	1 teaspoon

✦ ✦ ✦

Ravensara Aromatica	4 drops
Lavender	4 drops
Rosemary	2 drops
Cedarwood (*Atlas*)	2 drops
Carrier Oil	1 teaspoon

✦ ✦ ✦

Tea Tree	3 drops
Lavender	3 drops
Myrtle	3 drops
Leptospermum	3 drops
Carrier Oil	1 teaspoon

✦ ✦ ✦

Cypress	4 drops
Cabreuva	3 drops
Lemon	3 drops
Spruce	2 drops
Carrier Oil	1 teaspoon

DIFFUSOR

Place the oils in the glass bottle or on the pad, depending on the type of diffusor you have.

Peppermint	50%
Lavender	30%
Juniper	20%

✦ ✦ ✦

Spruce	40%
Lemon	30%
Eucalyptus	30%

✦ ✦ ✦

Cajeput	30%
Pine	30%
Cypress	30%
Orange	10%

✦ ✦ ✦

Juniper	30%
Spearmint	30%
Allspice	30%
Geranium	10%

MASSAGE

Massage into the upper chest, back of the neck, and shoulders until the oil is fully absorbed. Breathe in the vapors deeply.

Copaiba	5 drops
Spruce	4 drops
Myrtle	4 drops
Lovage	2 drops
Carrier Oil	1 tablespoon

✦ ✦ ✦

Lavender	4 drops
Spearmint	4 drops
Gingergrass	4 drops
Zanthoxylum	3 drops
Carrier Oil	1 tablespoon

✦ ✦ ✦

Leptospermum	4 drops
Eucalyptus	4 drops
Allspice	4 drops
Spearmint	3 drops
Carrier Oil	1 tablespoon

✦ ✦ ✦

Peppermint	5 drops
Marjoram	4 drops
Ravensara Aromatica	3 drops
Tea Tree	3 drops
Carrier Oil	1 tablespoon

MIST SPRAYS

Fill a fine mist spray bottle with purified water, then add essential oils. Tighten the cap, shake well, and mist numerous times over the head with eyes closed. Breathe in the vapors deeply.

Spearmint	60 drops
Lavender	60 drops
Cajeput	30 drops
Pure Water	4 ounces

✦ ✦ ✦

Spruce	50 drops
Leptospermum	50 drops
Eucalyptus Radiata	50 drops
Pure Water	4 ounces

STEAM INHALATION

Heat water and pour into a bowl, then add the essential oils. Immediately drape a towel over your head, close your eyes, and lean over towards the vapors. Inhale deeply.

Lavender	5 drops
Leptospermum	3 drops
Eucalyptus Radiata	2 drops

✦　　✦　　✦

Spruce	5 drops
Tangerine	3 drops
Cajeput	2 drops

✦　　✦　　✦

Hyssop Decumbens	4 drops
Tangerine	4 drops
Neroli	2 drops

✦　　✦　　✦

Spearmint	4 drops
Fennel	3 drops
Lavender	3 drops

CALMING

BATHS

Fill the bathtub with water as warm as you like. Mix the formula together, pour into the bathwater, and disperse the oil so that it is distributed evenly. Enjoy your bath for 30 minutes.

Leptospermum	5 drops
Cabreuva	5 drops
Neroli	5 drops
Carrier Oil	1 teaspoon

✦　　✦　　✦

Guaiacwood	5 drops
Zanthoxylum	5 drops
Champaca Flower	3 drops
Bois de Rose	2 drops
Carrier Oil	1 teaspoon

✦　　✦　　✦

Goldenrod	5 drops
Ylang-Ylang	4 drops
Monarda	4 drops
Tangerine	2 drops
Carrier Oil	1 teaspoon

✦　　✦　　✦

Clary Sage	4 drops
Sandalwood	4 drops
Elemi	4 drops
Champaca Flower	3 drops
Carrier Oil	1 teaspoon

DIFFUSOR

Place the oils in the glass bottle or on the pad, depending on the type of diffusor you have.

Bois de Rose	50%
Tangerine	50%

✦　　✦　　✦

Grapefruit	50%
Litsea Cubeba	30%
Cypress	20%

INHALER

Combine the essential oils into a small glass bottle and cap tightly. To use, inhale the vapors slowly and deeply fifteen to twenty times. Use whenever necessary.

Neroli	10 drops
Leptospermum	10 drops
Tangerine	10 drops

✦   ✦   ✦

Orange	25 drops
Vetiver	10 drops

MASSAGE

Massage into the upper chest, back of the neck, shoulders, and back until the oil is fully absorbed. Breathe in the vapors deeply.

Petitgrain	5 drops
Nutmeg	3 drops
Vetiver	3 drops
Vanilla	2 drops
Celery	2 drops
Carrier Oil	1 tablespoon

✦   ✦   ✦

Cedarwood (*Atlas*)	5 drops
Dill	4 drops
Tangerine	4 drops
Allspice	2 drops
Carrier Oil	1 tablespoon

✦   ✦   ✦

Monarda	5 drops
Chamomile (*Roman*)	5 drops
Clary Sage	3 drops
Bois de Rose	2 drops
Carrier Oil	1 tablespoon

✦   ✦   ✦

Amyris	5 drops
Rose	5 drops
Orange	5 drops
Carrier Oil	1 tablespoon

MIST SPRAYS

Fill a fine mist spray bottle with purified water, then add the essential oils. Tighten the cap, shake well, and mist numerous times over the head with eyes closed. Breathe in the vapors deeply.

Dill	50 drops
Orange	50 drops
Cabreuva	50 drops
Pure Water	4 ounces

✦   ✦   ✦

Elemi	40 drops
Lemongrass	40 drops
Ravensara Anisata	40 drops
Lavender	30 drops
Pure Water	4 ounces

CAR ALERT

Many car fatalities and injuries are caused by the driver falling asleep at the wheel. Fatigue is an especially common occurrence when driving long distances. It is always best not to drive if you are tired, but if you must drive, these formulas will help to keep you focused and alert.

INHALER

Combine the essential oils into a small glass bottle and cap tightly. To use, inhale the vapors slowly and deeply fifteen to twenty times. Use whenever necessary.

Peppermint	20 drops
Cinnamon Leaf	10 drops
Helichrysum	10 drops

✦   ✦   ✦

Spearmint	20 drops
Rosemary	10 drops
Cardamom	10 drops
Copaiba	10 drops

MIST SPRAYS

Fill a fine mist spray bottle with purified water, then add the essential oils. Tighten the cap, shake well, close the car windows, and mist numerous times into the car before driving. Breathe in the vapors deeply.

Peppermint	70 drops
Grapefruit	40 drops
Coriander	40 drops
Pure Water	4 ounces

✦ ✦ ✦

Spearmint	60 drops
Cardamom	30 drops
Lime	30 drops
Patchouli	30 drops
Pure Water	4 ounces

✦ ✦ ✦

Spearmint	60 drops
Helichrysum	35 drops
Cinnamon Leaf	30 drops
Patchouli	25 drops
Pure Water	4 ounces

✦ ✦ ✦

Rosemary	45 drops
Lemon	45 drops
Peppermint	40 drops
Copaiba	20 drops
Pure Water	4 ounces

DREAMS

These formulas are used to promote vivid dreams and clear recall. Apply one of the blends before bedtime. It is recommended that you repeat the application over a period of several nights.

MASSAGE

Massage into the upper chest, neck, and shoulder until the oil is fully absorbed.

Vanilla	3 drops
Lemon	3 drops
Sandalwood	2 drops
Basil (*Sweet*)	2 drops
Carrier Oil	2 teaspoons

✦ ✦ ✦

Orange	3 drops
Chamomile (*Roman*)	3 drops
Cinnamon Leaf	2 drops
Basil (*Sweet*)	2 drops
Carrier Oil	2 teaspoons

FACIAL CREME

Place the shea butter in a wide-mouthed glass jar and then put the jar in a small pot of water and heat on a low flame. When the shea butter has melted, add the sesame oil and stir. Remove the jar from the water and, as the ingredients cool, add the essential oils. Mix well. For best results, apply twice daily.

APPLICATION

Bois de Rose	20 drops
Sandalwood	10 drops
Shea Butter	4 teaspoons
Sesame	7 teaspoons

✦ ✦ ✦

Frankincense	10 drops
Tangerine	10 drops
Geranium	10 drops
Shea Butter	4 teaspoons
Sesame	7 teaspoons

HAIR CARE

Apply approximately 1 teaspoon of the blend into the scalp. Massage thoroughly into the scalp and hair until the oil has been absorbed.

APPLICATION

Copaiba	7 drops
Cedarwood (*Atlas*)	3 drops
Jojoba	1 tablespoon

✦   ✦   ✦

Bois de Rose	6 drops
Ginger	4 drops
Sesame	1 tablespoon

✦   ✦   ✦

Geranium	5 drops
Sandalwood	5 drops
Jojoba	1 tablespoon

✦   ✦   ✦

Copaiba	5 drops
Palmarosa	5 drops
Macadamia Nut	1 tablespoon

MENTAL CLARITY

BATHS

Fill the bathtub with water as warm as you like. Mix the formula together, pour into the bathwater, and disperse the oil so that it is distributed evenly. Enjoy your bath for 30 minutes.

Orange	4 drops
Hyssop Decumbens	4 drops
Rhododendron	4 drops
Ravensara Aromatica	3 drops
Carrier Oil	1 teaspoon

✦   ✦   ✦

Amyris	4 drops
Angelica Root	4 drops
Goldenrod	4 drops
Orange	3 drops
Carrier Oil	1 teaspoon

DIFFUSOR

Place the oils in the glass bottle or on the pad, depending on the type of diffusor you have.

Clove (*Bud*)	40%
Lime	30%
Petitgrain	30%

✦   ✦   ✦

Rosemary	30%
Juniper	25%
Lemon	25%
Clove (*Bud*)	20%

INHALER

Combine the essential oils into a small glass bottle and cap tightly. To use, inhale the vapors slowly and deeply fifteen to twenty times. Use whenever necessary.

Litsea Cubeba	10 drops
Hyssop Decumbens	10 drops
Lovage	5 drops

✦   ✦   ✦

Spearmint	15 drops
Basil (*Sweet*)	10 drops
Lemon	10 drops

MASSAGE

Massage into the upper chest, back of the neck, shoulders, and the back until the oil is fully absorbed.

Gingergrass	4 drops
Lime	4 drops
Pepper (*Black*)	4 drops
Sandalwood	3 drops
Carrier Oil	1 tablespoon

✦   ✦   ✦

Rosemary	4 drops
Peppermint	4 drops
Coriander	4 drops
Litsea Cubeba	3 drops
Carrier Oil	1 tablespoon

MIST SPRAYS

Fill a fine mist spray bottle with purified water and add the essential oils. Tighten the cap, shake well, and mist numerous times over the head with eyes closed. Breathe in the vapors deeply.

Peppermint	80 drops
Litsea Cubeba	50 drops
Patchouli	20 drops
Pure Water	4 ounces

✦　　✦　　✦

Cardamom	50 drops
Grapefruit	50 drops
Gingergrass	30 drops
Amyris	20 drops
Pure Water	4 ounces

MOOD UPLIFTING

DIFFUSOR

Place the oils in the glass bottle or on the pad, depending on the type of diffusor you have.

Juniper	25%
Cypress	25%
Orange	25%
Litsea Cubeba	25%

✦　　✦　　✦

Grapefruit	20%
Ravensara Anisata	20%
Spearmint	30%
Lavender	30%

INHALER

Combine the essential oils into a small glass bottle and cap tightly. To use, inhale the vapors slowly and deeply fifteen to twenty times. Use whenever necessary.

Vanilla	10 drops
Spearmint	10 drops
Petitgrain	10 drops

✦　　✦　　✦

Goldenrod	10 drops
Sandalwood	10 drops
Bois de Rose	10 drops

MASSAGE

Massage into the upper chest, back of the neck, shoulders, and the back until the oil is fully absorbed.

Champaca Flower	4 drops
Bois de Rose	4 drops
Orange	4 drops
Juniper	3 drops
Carrier Oil	1 tablespoon

✦　　✦　　✦

Cedarwood (*Atlas*)	5 drops
Neroli	4 drops
Vanilla	4 drops
Juniper	2 drops
Carrier Oil	1 tablespoon

MIST SPRAYS

Fill a fine mist spray bottle with purified water, then add the essential oils. Tighten the cap, shake well, and mist numerous times over the head with eyes closed. Breathe in the vapors deeply.

Orange	40 drops
Cinnamon Bark	30 drops
Grapefruit	30 drops
Cabreuva	20 drops
Pure Water	4 ounces

◆　　◆　　◆

Ylang-Ylang	40 drops
Amyris	40 drops
Rhododendron	20 drops
Mandarin	20 drops
Pure Water	4 ounces

MUSCLES; RELEASE TIGHTNESS

MASSAGE

Massage deeply into the specific muscles and the surrounding area(s) until the oil is fully absorbed.

Lavender	4 drops
Ginger	4 drops
Pepper (*Black*)	4 drops
Cabreuva	3 drops
Carrier Oil	1 tablespoon

◆　　◆　　◆

Allspice	5 drops
Leptospermum	5 drops
Marjoram	3 drops
Cabreuva	2 drops
Carrier Oil	1 tablespoon

NAIL CONDITIONER

Place the beeswax in a wide-mouthed glass jar and then put the jar in a small pot of water and heat on a low flame. When the beeswax has melted, add the carrier oil and stir. Remove the jar from the water and, as the ingredients cool, add the essential oils. Mix well.

Lemon	13 drops
Patchouli	7 drops
Beeswax	1 teaspoon
Carrier Oil	5 teaspoons

◆　　◆　　◆

Peppermint	7 drops
Fennel	7 drops
Bay (*West Indian*)	6 drops
Beeswax	1 teaspoon
Carrier Oil	5 teaspoons

ROMANCE

MASSAGE

Massage into the abdomen, upper chest, neck, shoulders, and back until the oil is fully absorbed.

Leptospermum	5 drops
Ambrette Seed	5 drops
Patchouli	4 drops
Cedarwood (*Atlas*)	3 drops
Vanilla	3 drops
Carrier Oil	4 teaspoons

◆　　◆　　◆

Geranium	5 drops
Labdanum	5 drops
Elemi	5 drops
Anise	3 drops
Sandalwood	2 drops
Carrier Oil	4 teaspoons

ROOM DISINFECTANT

DIFFUSOR

Place the oils in the glass bottle or on the pad, depending on the type of diffusor you have.

Cinnamon Bark	30%
Bergamot	30%
Rosemary	30%
Lemon	10%

✦ ✦ ✦

Eucalyptus	25%
Tea Tree	25%
Lavender	25%
Clove (*Bud*)	25%

MIST SPRAYS

Fill a fine mist spray bottle with purified water, then add the essential oils. Tighten the cap, shake well, and mist numerous times in the room.

Lavender	50 drops
Thyme	50 drops
Copaiba	30 drops
Cajeput	20 drops
Pure Water	4 ounces

✦ ✦ ✦

Lemon	50 drops
Clove (*Bud*)	50 drops
Tea Tree	30 drops
Patchouli	20 drops
Pure Water	4 ounces

SKIN CARE CREME

Place the shea butter in a wide-mouthed glass jar and then put the jar in a small pot of water and heat on a low flame. When the shea butter has melted, add the jojoba oil and stir. Remove the jar from the water and, as the ingredients cool, add the essential oils. Mix well. For best results, apply twice daily.

APPLICATION

Palmarosa	15 drops
Rose	15 drops
Litsea Cubeba	5 drops
Shea Butter	2 tablespoons
Jojoba	2 tablespoons

✦ ✦ ✦

Elemi	10 drops
Chamomile (*Roman*)	10 drops
Lavender	10 drops
Helichrysum	5 drops
Shea Butter	2 tablespoons
Jojoba	2 tablespoons

SLEEP RESTFULLY

MASSAGE

Massage into the upper chest, back of the neck, shoulders, and the back until the oil is fully absorbed. Use one of these formulas before going to sleep.

Vanilla	4 drops
Spikenard	4 drops
Rhododendron	2 drops
Carrier Oil	2 teaspoons

✦ ✦ ✦

Cabreuva	4 drops
Guaiacwood	4 drops
Tangerine	2 drops
Carrier Oil	2 teaspoons

STEAM AND SAUNA ROOM

Steam/sauna room with hot rocks: Fill a container with water, then add the essential oils and stir. Pour over the hot rocks and enjoy the aroma.

Eucalyptus	5 drops
Lavender	5 drops
Container of Water	

✦   ✦   ✦

Spearmint	8 drops
Sandalwood	2 drops
Container of Water	

✦   ✦   ✦

Cedarwood (*Atlas*)	5 drops
Cypress	5 drops
Container of Water	

✦   ✦   ✦

Myrtle	5 drops
Spruce	5 drops
Container of Water	

✦   ✦   ✦

Ravensara Aromatica	5 drops
Cajeput	5 drops
Container of Water	

✦   ✦   ✦

Tea Tree	5 drops
Fennel	5 drops
Container of Water	

MIST SPRAYS

Fill a fine mist spray bottle with purified water, then add the essential oils. Tighten the cap, shake well, and mist numerous times away from your body and face to ensure that the oil particles do not come in direct contact with your skin or eyes, since the oils can become very irritating to the skin, especially in the hot steam and sauna room.

Fir Needles	50 drops
Spruce	50 drops
Cedarwood (*Atlas*)	20 drops
Pure Water	4 ounces

✦   ✦   ✦

Leptospermum	50 drops
Eucalyptus Radiata	50 drops
Ravensara Anisata	20 drops
Pure Water	4 ounces

STRESS-FREE

BATHS

Fill the bathtub with water as warm as you like. Mix the formula together, pour into the bathwater, and disperse the oil so that it is distributed evenly. Enjoy your bath for 30 minutes.

Leptospermum	4 drops
Lavender	4 drops
Cabreuva	4 drops
Orange	2 drops
Carrier Oil	1 teaspoon

✦   ✦   ✦

Copaiba	4 drops
Mandarin	4 drops
Cypress	3 drops
Ravensara Anisata	3 drops
Carrier Oil	1 teaspoon

INHALER

Combine the essential oils into a small glass bottle and cap tightly. To use, inhale the vapors slowly and deeply fifteen to twenty times. Use whenever necessary.

Vetiver	10 drops
Litsea Cubeba	10 drops
Orange	10 drops

✦   ✦   ✦

Bergamot	10 drops
Geranium	10 drops
Spikenard	10 drops

MASSAGE

Massage into the abdomen, upper chest, back of the neck, shoulders, and the back until the oil is fully absorbed. In addition, massaging the bottoms of the feet will help to alleviate stress.

Labdanum	5 drops
Lemongrass	5 drops
Guaiacwood	5 drops
Elemi	5 drops
Carrier Oil	4 teaspoons

✦   ✦   ✦

Clary Sage	4 drops
Lime	4 drops
Zanthoxylum	4 drops
Allspice	4 drops
Sandalwood	4 drops
Carrier Oil	4 teaspoons

MIST SPRAYS

Fill a fine mist spray bottle with purified water, then add the essential oils. Tighten the cap, shake well, and mist numerous times over the head with eyes closed. Breathe in the vapors deeply.

Spearmint	50 drops
Ravensara Anisata	30 drops
Amyris	30 drops
Leptospermum	20 drops
Clove (*Bud*)	20 drops
Pure Water	4 ounces

✦   ✦   ✦

Mandarin	30 drops
Lime	30 drops
Amyris	30 drops
Grapefruit	30 drops
Chamomile (*Roman*)	30 drops
Pure Water	4 ounces

WARMING

MASSAGE

Massage into the upper chest, back of the neck, shoulders, and hands and feet until the oil is fully absorbed into the skin.

Ginger	4 drops
Goldenrod	4 drops
Copaiba	4 drops
Thyme	3 drops
Carrier Oil	1 tablespoon

✦   ✦   ✦

Cardamom	4 drops
Zanthoxylum	4 drops
Marjoram	4 drops
Ravensara Anisata	3 drops
Carrier Oil	1 tablespoon

CHAPTER 7

Category Listings of Oil Properties

MOOD UPLIFTING

Allspice
Ambrette Seed
Amyris
Basil (*Sweet*)
Benzoin
Bergamot
Birch
Bois de Rose
Cabreuva
Calamint
Camphor
Cananga
Cardamom
Carnation
Cascarilla Bark
Cassia
Cassie
Chamomile
Champaca Flower
Cinnamon
Citronella
Clary Sage
Clove
Coffee
Copaiba
Cornmint
Cumin
Cypress
Elecampane
Elemi
Fir Balsam Needles
Fir Balsam Resin
Fir Needles
Frankincense
Galangal
Galbanum
Gardenia
Geranium
Ginger
Gingergrass
Goldenrod
Grapefruit
Helichrysum
Hyssop
Jasmine
Juniper
Labdanum
Lantana
Larch
Lavandin
Lavender
Lemon
Lemon Verbena
Lemongrass
Leptospermum
Lime
Litsea Cubeba
Lovage
Mandarin
Massoia Bark
Melissa
Mimosa
Monarda
Myrrh
Myrtle
Neroli
Nutmeg
Orange
Oregano
Palmarosa
Patchouli
Peppermint
Peru Balsam
Petitgrain
Pine
Ravensara Anisata
Ravensara Aromatica
Rhododendron
Rose
Rosemary
Sandalwood
Spearmint
Spikenard
Spruce
Spruce-Hemlock
St. John's Wort
Styrax
Tangelo
Tangerine
Tea Tree
Temple Orange
Thyme
Tolu Balsam
Turmeric
Vanilla
Vetiver
Violet
Ylang-Ylang
Zanthoxylum

ENERGIZING, REFRESHING, REVIVING

Some oils can be reviving to one person and calming to another. This is due to an adaptogen property that the oil has to bring balance to the body.

Amyris
Bergamot
Camphor
Cardamom
Cassia
Cinnamon
Citronella
Clove
Coffee
Coriander
Cornmint
Cumin
Cypress
Eucalyptus
Eucalyptus Citriodora
Fir Balsam Needles
Fir Needles
Galangal
Geranium
Ginger
Grapefruit
Helichrysum

Hyssop
Juniper
Lemon
Lemon Verbena
Lemongrass
Lime
Litsea Cubeba
Massoia Bark
Myrtle
Nutmeg
Oregano

Palmarosa
Pepper (*Black*)
Peppermint
Pine
Ravensara Aromatica
Rosemary
Spearmint
Tea Tree
Terebinth
Thyme

Mugwort
Myrrh
Myrtle
Neroli
Nutmeg
Orange
Palmarosa
Parsley
Peru Balsam
Petitgrain
Ravensara Anisata
Ravensara Aromatica
Rhododendron
Rose
Sage
Sandalwood
Spikenard

Spruce
Spruce-Hemlock
St. John's Wort
Styrax
Tangelo
Tangerine
Temple Orange
Tobacco
Turmeric
Valerian
Vanilla
Vetiver
Violet
Yarrow
Ylang-Ylang
Zanthoxylum

CALMING/STRESS REDUCING

Allspice
Ambrette Seed
Amyris
Angelica
Anise
Basil (*Sweet*)
Bay (*Sweet*)
Bay (*West Indian*)
Benzoin
Bergamot
Birch
Bois de Rose
Cabreuva
Cajeput
Calamint
Cananga
Cascarilla Bark
Cedarwood
Celery
Chamomile
Champaca Flower
Champaca Leaf
Cinnamon
Citronella
Clary Sage
Copaiba
Costus
Cumin
Cyperus
Cypress
Dill
Elemi
Eucalyptus Citriodora

Eucalyptus Radiata
Fennel
Fir Balsam Needles
Fir Balsam Resin
Fir Needles
Frankincense
Galangal
Galbanum
Geranium
Gingergrass
Goldenrod
Grapefruit
Guaiacwood
Helichrysum
Hops
Juniper
Labdanum
Lantana
Lavandin
Lavender
Ledum Groenlandicum
Lemon
Lemongrass
Leptospermum
Lime
Linden Blossom
Litsea Cubeba
Lovage
Mandarin
Marjoram
Massoia Bark
Melissa
Monarda

PROMOTES A RESTFUL SLEEP

Ajowan
Allspice
Anise
Basil (*Sweet*)
Benzoin
Bergamot
Birch
Cajeput
Cananga
Cedarwood
Celery
Chamomile
Clary Sage
Copaiba
Costus
Cyperus
Cypress
Dill
Elemi
Fennel
Fir Balsam Resin
Frankincense
Guaiacwood
Hops
Labdanum
Lantana

Lavandin
Lavender
Lemon
Lemongrass
Linden Blossom
Litsea Cubeba
Mandarin
Marjoram
Melissa
Myrrh
Neroli
Nutmeg
Orange
Peru Balsam
Petitgrain
Ravensara Anisata
Sandalwood
Spikenard
Spruce
Spruce-Hemlock
Styrax
Tangelo
Tangerine
Temple Orange
Turmeric
Valerian

Vanilla
Vetiver
Violet
Ylang-Ylang
Zanthoxylum

VAPORS OPEN THE BREATHING

Allspice
Angelica
Anise
Bay (*Sweet*)
Bay (*West Indian*)
Cajeput
Camphor
Cedarwood
Clove
Cornmint
Cubeb
Eucalyptus
Eucalyptus Citriodora
Fir Balsam Needles
Fir Needles
Gingergrass
Helichrysum
Hyssop
Larch
Lavandin
Lavender
Lemongrass
Marjoram
Mastic
Myrtle
Niaouli
Oregano
Peppermint
Pine
Ravensara Anisata
Ravensara Aromatica
Rosemary
Spearmint
Spruce
Spruce-Hemlock
Tea Tree
Terebinth
Thyme
Yarrow
Zanthoxylum

MENTAL CLARITY

Amyris
Angelica
Basil (*Sweet*)
Bay (*Sweet*)
Bay (*West Indian*)
Bergamot
Cabreuva
Calamint
Cardamom
Cedarwood (*Atlas*)
Champaca Leaf
Citronella
Clove
Coffee
Copaiba
Coriander
Cornmint
Cypress
Eucalyptus
Fir Balsam Needles
Fir Needles
Ginger
Gingergrass
Goldenrod
Grapefruit
Guaiacwood
Helichrysum
Hyssop
Juniper
Ledum Groenlandicum
Lemon
Lemon Verbena
Leptospermum
Lime
Litsea Cubeba
Lovage

Mandarin
Massoia Bark
Monarda
Nutmeg
Orange
Oregano
Pepper (*Black*)
Peppermint
Petitgrain
Pine
Ravensara Anisata
Ravensara Aromatica
Rhododendron
Rosemary
Spearmint
Spruce
Spruce-Hemlock
St. John's Wort
Tangelo
Tangerine
Tarragon
Tea Tree
Temple Orange
Terebinth
Thyme
Turmeric
Yarrow
Zanthoxylum

IMPROVES DIGESTION

Allspice
Angelica
Anise
Basil (*Sweet*)
Bay (*Sweet*)
Bay (*West Indian*)
Caraway
Cardamom
Chamomile
Cinnamon
Clary Sage
Clove
Coriander
Cornmint
Cubeb
Cumin
Dill
Fennel
Galangal
Ginger
Lavandin
Lavender
Lemongrass
Litsea Cubeba
Marjoram
Nutmeg
Oregano
Parsley
Pepper (*Black*)
Peppermint
Rosemary
Sage
Spearmint
Thyme
Vetiver

COOLING

Amyris
Angelica
Basil (*Sweet*)
Bergamot
Cedarwood (*Atlas*)
Celery
Citronella
Cornmint
Costus
Eucalyptus
Geranium
Grapefruit
Helichrysum
Lantana

Lemon
Lime
Litsea Cubeba
Mandarin
Myrrh
Orange
Peppermint

Petitgrain
Rose
Spearmint
Tangelo
Tangerine
Temple Orange

WARMING/HEATING

Allspice
Bay (*Sweet*)
Bay (*West Indian*)
Benzoin
Birch (*Sweet*)
Cabreuva
Cajeput
Cardamom
Cascarilla Bark
Cassia
Champaca Flower
Champaca Leaf
Cinnamon
Clove
Coffee
Copaiba
Cumin
Cyperus
Elemi
Fennel

Fir Balsam Resin
Ginger
Gingergrass
Goldenrod
Labdanum
Ledum Groenlandicum
Marjoram
Massoia Bark
Nutmeg
Oregano
Palmarosa
Pepper (*Black*)
Peru Balsam
Ravensara Anisata
Rosemary
Savory
Turmeric
Thyme
Zanthoxylum

LESSENS OR RELIEVES PAIN

Allspice
Aloe Vera
Ambrette Seed
Angelica
Anise
Arnica
Basil (*Sweet*)
Bay (*Sweet*)
Bay (*West Indian*)
Birch
Bois de Rose
Cabreuva
Cade
Cajeput

Calamint
Cananga
Caraway
Cardamom
Cassia
Cedarwood
Chamomile
Cinnamon
Clary Sage
Clove
Coriander
Cornmint
Cubeb
Cumin

Dill
Eucalyptus
Fennel
Fir Balsam Needles
Fir Needles
Galangal
Galbanum
Geranium
Ginger
Goldenrod
Helichrysum
Hops
Juniper
Lavandin
Lavender
Leptospermum
Litsea Cubeba
Marjoram
Melissa
Myrtle
Niaouli
Nutmeg

Oregano
Palmarosa
Peppermint
Pine
Ravensara Anisata
Ravensara Aromatica
Rose
Rosemary
Rue
Sage
Sassafras
Savory
Spearmint
St. John's Wort
Tarragon
Tea Tree
Terebinth
Thyme
Valerian
Vetiver
Ylang-Ylang

HEALING TO THE SKIN

Aloe Vera
Ambrette Seed
Arnica
Benzoin
Bois de Rose
Calendula
Chamomile
Cocoa Butter
Copaiba
Elemi
Frankincense
Lavandin
Lavender

Leptospermum
Mangosteen
Myrrh
Palmarosa
Patchouli
Peru Balsam
Rose
Sandalwood
Tagetes
Tea Tree
Vegetal/Carrier Oils
Vetiver

REDUCES CELLULITE

Allspice
Basil (*Sweet*)
Bay (*Sweet*)
Bay (*West Indian*)
Benzoin

Bergamot
Birch
Cassia
Celery
Cinnamon

Cumin
Cypress
Fennel
Fir Balsam Needles
Fir Balsam Resin
Fir Needles
Geranium
Grapefruit
Juniper
Lavandin
Lavender
Lemon
Lime

Lovage
Mandarin
Orange
Oregano
Pine
Rosemary
Sage
Sassafras
Styrax
Tangelo
Tangerine
Temple Orange
Thyme

INSECT BITES

Aloe Vera
Basil (*Sweet*)
Calendula
Chamomile
Fir Balsam Resin
Geranium

Juniper
Lavandin
Lavender
Lemon
Lime
Tea Tree

INSECT REPELLENT

Bay (*Sweet*)
Bay (*West Indian*)
Cajeput
Cassia
Cedarwood
Cinnamon
Citronella
Clove
Cornmint
Dill
Eucalyptus
Fennel
Geranium

Juniper
Lavandin
Lavender
Lemongrass
Oregano
Patchouli
Pennyroyal
Peppermint
Rosemary
Spearmint
Terebinth
Thyme
Vetiver

AVOID DURING PREGNANCY

Allspice
Aloe Vera
Anise
Arnica
Basil (*Sweet*)

Bay (*Sweet*)
Bay (*West Indian*)
Calendula
Camphor
Caraway

Carrot
Cassia
Cedarwood
Celery
Cinnamon
Clary Sage
Clove
Fennel
Hops
Hyssop
Juniper
Labdanum
Lemon Verbena
Lovage
Marjoram
Mugwort
Myrrh
Nutmeg

Oregano
Parsley
Pennyroyal
Pepper (*Black*)
Peppermint
Rosemary
Rue
Sage
Savory
Sassafras
Spikenard
St. John's Wort
Tarragon
Thyme
Valerian
Wormwood
Yarrow

PERMISSIBLE DURING PREGNANCY

Use only in small amounts—2 to 3 drops of an oil per application.

Bergamot
Cananga
Coriander
Cypress
Frankincense
Geranium
Ginger
Grapefruit
Lavandin
Lavender
Lemon
Mandarin

Neroli
Orange
Patchouli
Petitgrain
Sandalwood
Spearmint
Tangelo
Tangerine
Tea Tree
Temple Orange
Ylang-Ylang

A Cross-Reference of Botanical Names

❧❧❧

Abelmoschus moschatus—Ambrette Seed

Abies alba—Fir Needles, Silver Fir

Abies balsamea—Fir Balsam Needles, Fir Balsam Resin

Abies balsamifera—Fir Balsam Resin

Abies grandis—Grand Fir, Fir Needles

Acacia dealbata—Mimosa

Acacia decurrens—Mimosa

Acacia farnesiana—Cassie

Achillea millefolium—Yarrow

Acorus calamus—Calamus (*Sweet Flag*)

Actinidia chinensis—Kiwifruit Seed

Aleurites moluccana—Kukui Nut

Aloe barbadensis—Aloe Vera

Aloysia citriodora—Lemon Verbena

Aloysia triphylla—Lemon Verbena

Alpinia officinarum—Galangal

Amomoum curcuma—Turmeric

Amyris balsamifera—Amyris

Anacardium occidentale—Cashew Nut

Andropogon martinii—Palmarosa

Andropogon muricatus—Vetiver

Andropogon nardus—Citronella

Anethum foeniculum—Fennel

Anethum graveolens—Dill

Angelica archangelica—Angelica

Angelica levisticum—Lovage

Angelica officinalis—Angelica

Aniba rosaeodora—Bois de Rose (*Rosewood*)

Anisum officinalis—Anise

Anthemis mixta—Chamomile (*Moroccan*)

Anthemis nobilis—Chamomile (*Roman*)

Apium carvi—Caraway

Apium graveolens—Celery

Apium petroselinum—Parsley

Arachis hypogaea—Peanut

Armeniaca vulgaris—Apricot Kernel

Arnica montana—Arnica

Artemisia absinthium—Wormwood

Artemisia dracunculus—Tarragon (*Estragon*)

Artemisia vulgaris—Mugwort (*Armoise*)

Aster officinalis—Elecampane

Azadirachta indica—Neem

Balsam styracis—Styrax

Balsamodendrom myrrha—Myrrh

Baryosma tongo—Tonka Bean (*Tonquin Bean*)

Bertholletia excelsa—Brazil Nut

Betula alba—Birch (*White*)

Betula capinefolia—Birch (*Sweet*)

Betula lenta—Birch (*Sweet*)

Borago officinalis—Borage

Boswellia carteri—Frankincense (*Olibanum*)

Boswellia thurifera—Frankincense (*Olibanum*)

Brassica napus—Canola (*Rapeseed*)

Bulnesia sarmienti—Guaiacwood

Butyrosperum parkii—Shea Butter

Calamintha clinopodium—Calamint (*Catnip*)

Calamintha hortensis—Savory

Calamintha officinalis—Calamint (*Catnip*)

Calamus aromaticus—Calamus (*Sweet Flag*)

Calendula officinalis—Calendula (*Marigold*)

Calophyllum inophyllum—Calophyllum

Camellia japonica—Camellia

Cananga odorata—Cananga

Cananga odorata var. *genuina*—Ylang-Ylang

Canarium commune—Elemi

Canarium luzonicum—Elemi

Carthamus tinctorius—Safflower

Carum carvi—Caraway

Carum petroselinum—Parsley

Carya illinoinensis—Pecan

Cassia ancienne—Cassie

Cedrus atlantica—Cedarwood (*Atlas*)

Chamaemelum nobile—Chamomile (*Roman*)

Cinnamomum aromaticum—Cassia

Cinnamomum camphora—Camphor, Ravensara Anisata, Ravensara Aromatica

Cinnamomum cassia—Cassia

Cinnamomum vera—Cinnamon

Cinnamomum zeylanicum—Cinnamon

Cistus ladanifer—Labdanum (*Cistus* or Rock Rose)
Citrus aurantiifolia—Lime
Citrus aurantium—Neroli, Orange (*Bitter*)
Citrus bergamia—Bergamot
Citrus bigaradia—Petitgrain
Citrus limetta—Lime
Citrus limon—Lemon
Citrus madurensis—Mandarin
Citrus nobilis—Mandarin
Citrus paradisi—Grapefruit
Citrus racemosa—Grapefruit
Citrus reticulata—Mandarin, Tangerine, Temple Orange
Citrus sinensis—Orange (*Sweet*)
Citrus tangelo—Tangelo
Cocos nucifera—Coconut
Coffea arabica—Coffee
Commiphora myrrha—Myrrh
Copaifera officinalis—Copaiba
Coriandrum sativum—Coriander
Corylus avellana—Hazelnut
Coumarouna odorata—Tonka Bean (*Tonquin Bean*)
Crocus sativus—Saffron
Croton eleuteria—Cascarilla Bark
Cryptocarya massoia—Massoia Bark
Cubeba officinalis—Cubeb
Cucurbita pepo—Pumpkinseed
Cuminum cyminum—Cumin
Cuminum odorum—Cumin
Cupressus sempervirens—Cypress
Curcuma domestica—Turmeric
Curcuma longa—Turmeric
Cymbopogon citratus—Lemongrass
Cymbopogon flexuosus—Lemongrass
Cymbopogon martinii var. *motia*—Palmarosa
Cymbopogon martinii var. *sofia*—Gingergrass
Cymbopogon nardus—Citronella
Cyperus scariosus—Cyperus (*Cypriol*)
Daucus carota—Carrot (*Root* or *Seed*)
Dianthus caryophyllus—Carnation (*Clove Pink*)
Dipteryx odorata—Tonka Bean (*Tonquin Bean*)
Dryobalanops aromatica—Camphor (*Borneol*)
Dryobalanops camphora—Camphor (*Borneol*)
Elaeis guineensis—Palm & Palm Kernel
Elettaria cardamomum—Cardamom

Eucalyptus citriodora—Eucalyptus Citriodora
Eucalyptus globulus—Eucalyptus
Eucalyptus radiata—Eucalyptus Radiata
Eugenia aromatica—Clove
Eugenia caryophyllata—Clove
Eugenia caryophyllus—Clove
Fagus grandifolia—Beechnut
Fagus sylvatica—Beechnut
Ferula galbaniflua—Galbanum
Ferula gummosa—Galbanum
Ferula rubicaulis—Galbanum
Foeniculum officinale—Fennel
Foeniculum vulgare—Fennel
Fructus anethi—Dill
Garcinia mangostana—Mangosteen (*Kokum Butter*)
Gardenia grandiflora—Gardenia
Gaultheria procumbens—Wintergreen
Gossypium species—Cottonseed
Guaiacum officinale—Guaiacwood
Helenium grandiflorum—Elecampane
Helianthus annuus—Sunflower
Helichrysum angustifolium—Helichrysum (*Everlasting* or *Immortelle*)
Helichrysum italicum—Helichrysum (*Everlasting* or *Immortelle*)
Hibiscus abelmoschus—Ambrette Seed
Hippophae rhamnoides—Sea Buckthorn
Humulus lupulus—Hops
Hydnocarpus kurzii—Chaulmoogra
Hydnocarpus laurifolia—Chaulmoogra
Hypericum perforatum—St. John's Wort
Hyssopus officinalis—Hyssop
Hyssopus officinalis var. *decumbens*—Hyssop Decumbens
Illicium verum—Anise (*Star*)
Inula helenium—Elecampane
Iris florentina—Orris Root
Iris pallida—Orris Root
Jasminum officinale—Jasmine
Juglans regia—Walnut
Juniperus communis—Juniper Berries
Juniperus oxycedrus—Cade
Juniperus virginiana—Cedarwood
Languas officinarum—Galangal
Lantana camara—Lantana
Larix europaea—Larch

Laurus camphora—Camphor
Laurus cassia—Cassia
Laurus cinnamomum—Cinnamon
Laurus nobilis—Bay (*Sweet*)
Lavandula augustifolia—Lavender
Lavandula fragrans—Lavandin
Lavandula hortensis—Lavandin
Lavandula hybrida—Lavandin
Lavandula officinalis—Lavender
Lavandula taemina—Santolina
Lavandula vera—Lavender
Ledum groenlandicum—Ledum Groenlandicum
Leptospermum citratum—Leptospermum (*New Zealand Tea Tree*)
Leptospermum ericoides (Kanuka)—Leptospermum (*New Zealand Tea Tree*)
Leptospermum petersonii—Leptospermum (*New Zealand Tea Tree*)
Leptospermum scoparium—Leptospermum (*New Zealand Tea Tree*)
Levisticum officinale—Lovage
Ligusticum levisticum—Lovage
Linum usitatissimum—Flaxseed
Lippia citriodora—Lemon Verbena
Lippia triphylla—Lemon Verbena
Liquidamber orientalis—Styrax (*Liquidamber* or *Storax*)
Liquidamber styraciflua—Styrax (*Liquidamber* or *Storax*)
Litsea citrata—Litsea Cubeba
Litsea cubeba—Litsea Cubeba
Macadamia integrifolia—Macadamia Nut
Majorana hortensis—Marjoram (*Sweet*)
Mangifera indica—Mango
Matricaria chamomilla—Chamomile (*German*)
Matricaria recutica—Chamomile (*German*)
Melaleuca alternifolia—Tea Tree
Melaleuca cajuputi—Cajeput
Melaleuca leucadendron—Cajeput
Melaleuca linariifolia—Tea Tree
Melaleuca minor—Cajeput
Melaleuca quinquenervia—Niaouli
Melaleuca uncinata—Tea Tree
Melaleuca viridiflora—Niaouli
Melissa officinalis—Melissa (*Lemon Balm*)
Mentha arvensis—Cornmint
Mentha piperita—Peppermint

Mentha pulegium—Pennyroyal
Mentha spicata—Spearmint
Mentha virdis—Spearmint
Michelia alba—Champaca
Michelia champaca—Champaca
Monarda fistulosa—Monarda
Moringa oleifera—Ben
Moringa pterygosperma—Ben
Myrcia acris—Bay (*West Indian*)
Myristica aromata—Nutmeg
Myristica fragrans—Nutmeg
Myristica officinalis—Nutmeg
Myrocarpus fastigiatus—Cabreuva
Myrosperum pereira—Peru Balsam
Myroxylon balsamum—Tolu Balsam
Myroxylon pereirae—Peru Balsam
Myrtus communis—Myrtle
Nardostachys jatamansi—Spikenard
Nepeta cataria—Calamint (*Catnip*)
Nicotiana tabacum—Tobacco Leaf
Ocimum basilicum—Basil (*Sweet*)
Oenothera biennis—Evening Primrose
Olea europaea—Olive
Oncoba echinata—Chaulmoogra
Orbignya barbosiana—Babassu
Origanum majorana—Marjoram (*Sweet*)
Origanum vulgare—Oregano
Ormenis mixta—Chamomile (*Moroccan*)
Ormenis multicaulis—Chamomile (*Moroccan*)
Oryza sativa—Rice Bran
Osmanthus fragrans—Osmanthus
Passiflora incarnata—Passion Fruit Seed
Pelargonium graveolens—Geranium
Persea americana—Avocado
Persea gratissima—Avocado
Petroselinum hortense—Parsley
Petroselinum sativum—Parsley
Peucedanum graveolens—Dill
Picea mariana—Spruce
Picea sitchensis—Spruce-Sitka
Pimenta acris—Bay (*West Indian*)
Pimenta dioica—Allspice
Pimenta officinalis—Allspice
Pimenta racemosa—Bay (*West Indian*)
Pimpinella anisum—Anise
Pinus balsaamea—Fir Balsam Resin
Pinus edulis—Pine Nut

Pinus maritima—Terebinth
Pinus palustris—Terebinth
Pinus pinea—Pine Nut
Pinus sylvestris—Pine
Piper cubeba—Cubeb
Piper nigrum—Pepper (*Black*)
Pistacia lentiscus—Mastic
Pistacia terebinthus—Terebinth
Pistacia vera—Pistachio Nut
Pogostemon cablin—Patchouli
Pogostemon patchouli—Patchouli
Polianthes tuberosa—Tuberose
Prunus amygdalus—Almond (*Sweet*)
Prunus armeniaca—Apricot Kernel
Prunus dulcis—Almond (*Sweet*)
Pseudotsuga menziesii—Douglas Fir
Ravensara anisata—Ravensara Anisata (*Havozo Bark*)
Ravensara aromatica—Ravensara Aromatica
Rhododendron anthopogon—Rhododendron
Ribes nigrum—Black Currant Seed
Ricinus communis—Castor
Rosa centifolia—Rose
Rosa damascena—Rose
Rosa rubiginosa—Rose Hip Seed
Rosmarinus coronarium—Rosemary
Rosmarinus officinalis—Rosemary
Ruta graveolens—Rue
Salvia lavandulifolia—Sage (*Spanish*)
Salvia officinalis—Sage
Salvia sclarea—Clary Sage
Santalum album—Sandalwood
Santolina chamaecyparissus—Santolina (*Lavender Cotton*)
Sassafras albidum—Sassafras
Satureja calamintha—Calamint (*Catnip*)
Satureja hortensis—Savory
Satureja montana—Savory
Saussurea costus—Costus
Saussurea lappa—Costus
Schimmelia oleifera—Amyris
Sesamum indicum—Sesame
Simmondsia chinensis—Jojoba

Sisymbrium officinale—Sisymbrium
Soja hispida—Soybean
Solidago canadensis—Goldenrod
Solidago odora—Goldenrod
Styrax benzoin—Benzoin
Styrax tonkinensis—Benzoin
Syzygium aromaticum—Clove
Tagetes erecta—Tagetes
Tagetes minuta—Tagetes
Tagetes patula—Tagetes
Taraktagenos kurzii—Chaulmoogra
Theobroma cacao—Cocoa Butter
Thuja occidentalis—Thuja (*Cedar Leaf*)
Thymus aestivus—Thyme
Thymus citriodora—Thyme
Thymus ilerdensis—Thyme
Thymus mastichina—Marjoram (*Spanish*)
Thymus satureiodes—Thyme
Thymus valentianus—Thyme
Thymus vulgaris—Thyme
Thymus vulgaris var. *linalol*—Thyme Linalol
Thymus webbianus—Thyme
Tilia europaea—Linden Blossom
Tilia vulgaris—Linden Blossom
Toluifera pereira—Peru Balsam
Trachyspermum ammi—Ajowan
Trachyspermum copticum—Ajowan
Triticum vulgare—Wheat Germ
Tsuga canadensis—Spruce-Hemlock
Unona odorantissimum—Ylang-Ylang
Valeriana officinalis—Valerian
Vanilla fragrans—Vanilla
Vanilla planifolia—Vanilla
Verbena triphylla—Lemon Verbena
Vetiveria zizanoides—Vetiver
Viola odorata—Violet
Vitis vinifera—Grapeseed
Zanthoxylum alatum—Zanthoxylum
Zanthoxylum americanum—Zanthoxylum
Zanthoxylum rhesta—Zanthoxylum
Zea mays—Corn
Zingiber officinale—Ginger

Plant Family Name Classification

Actinidiaceae

Kiwifruit Seed—*Actinidia chinensis*

Agavaceae

Tuberose—*Polianthes tuberosa*

Anacardiaceae

Cashew Nut—*Anacardium occidentale*
Mango—*Mangifera indica*
Mastic—*Pistacia lentiscus*
Pistachio Nut—*Pistacia vera*
Terebinth—*Pistacia terebinthus*

Annonaceae

Cananga—*Cananga odorata*
Ylang-Ylang—*Cananga odorata* var. *genuina*,
    Unona odorantissimum

Apiaceae

Ajowan—*Trachyspermum ammi, T. copticum*
Angelica—*Angelica archangelica, A. officinalis*
Anise—*Anisum officinalis, Pimpinella anisum*
Caraway—*Apium carvi, Carum carvi*
Carrot—*Daucus carota*
Celery—*Apium graveolens*
Coriander—*Coriandrum sativum*
Cumin—*Cuminum cyminum, C. odorum*
Dill—*Anethum graveolens, Fructus anethi,*
    Peucedanum graveolens
Fennel—*Anethum foeniculum, Foeniculum*
    officinale, F. vulgare
Galbanum—*Ferula galbaniflua, F. gummosa,*
    F. rubicaulis
Lovage—*Angelica levisticum, Levisticum*
    officinale, Ligusticum levisticum
Parsley—*Apium petroselinum, Carum*
    petroselinum, Petroselinum hortense, P. sativum

Araceae

Calamus (*Sweet Flag*)—*Acorus calamus, Calamus*
    aromaticus

Arecaceae

Babassu—*Orbignya barbosiana*
Coconut—*Cocus nucifera*
Palm—*Elaeis guineensis*

Asteraceae

Arnica—*Arnica montana*
Calendula (*Marigold*)—*Calendula officinalis*
Chamomile (*German*)—*Matricaria chamomilla,*
    M. recutica
Chamomile (*Moroccan*)—*Anthemis mixta,*
    Ormenis mixta, O. multicaulis
Chamomile (*Roman*)—*Anthemis nobilis,*
    Chamaemelum nobile
Costus—*Saussurea costus, S. lappa*
Elecampane—*Aster officinalis, Helenium grandi-*
    florum, Inula helenium
Goldenrod—*Solidago canadensis, S. odora*
Helichrysum (*Everlasting* or *Immortelle*)—
    Helichrysum angustifolium, H. italicum
Mugwort (*Armoise*)—*Artemisia vulgaris*
Safflower—*Carthamus tinctorius*
Santolina (*Lavender Cotton*)—*Lavandula taemi-*
    na, Santolina chamaecyparissus
Sunflower—*Helianthus annuus*
Tagetes—*Tagetes erecta, T. minuta, T. patula*
Tarragon (*Estragon*)—*Artemisia dracunculus*
Wormwood—*Artemisia absinthium*
Yarrow—*Achillea millefolium*

Betulaceae

Birch (*Sweet*)—*Betula capinefolia, B. lenta*
Birch (*White*)—*Betula alba*
Hazelnut—*Corylus avellana*

Boraginaceae

Borage—*Borage officinalis*

Brassicaceae

Canola (*Rapeseed*)—*Brassica napus*
Sisymbrium (*Hedge Mustard*)—*Sisymbrium officinale*

Burseraceae

Elemi—*Canarium commune, C. luzonicum*
Frankincense (*Olibanum*)—*Boswellia carteri, B. thurifera*
Myrrh—*Balsamodendrom myrrha, Commiphora myrrha*

Buxaceae

Jojoba—*Simmondsia chinensis*

Caryophyllaceae

Carnation (*Clove Pink*)—*Dianthus caryophyllus*

Cistaceae

Labdanum (*Cistus* or *Rock Rose*)—*Cistus ladanifer*

Cucurbitaceae

Pumpkinseed—*Cucurbita pepo*

Cupressaceae

Cade—*Juniperus oxycedrus*
Cedarwood—*Juniperus virginiana*
Cypress—*Cupressus sempervirens*
Juniper Berries—*Juniperus communis*
Thuja (*Cedar Leaf*)—*Thuja occidentalis*

Cyperaceae

Cyperus (*Cypriol*)—*Cyperus scariosus*

Dipterocarpaceae

Camphor (*Borneol*)—*Dryobalanops aromatica, D. camphora*

Elaeagnaceae

Sea Buckthorn—*Hippophae rhamnoides*

Ericaceae

Ledum Groenlandicum—*Ledum groenlandicum*
Rhododendron—*Rhododendron anthopogon*
Wintergreen—*Gaultheria procumbens*

Euphorbiaceae

Cascarilla Bark—*Croton eleuteria*
Castor—*Ricinus communis*
Kukui Nut—*Aleurites moluccana*

Fabaceae

Cabreuva—*Myrocarpus fastigiatus*
Copaiba—*Copaifera officinalis*
Peanut—*Arachis hypogaea*
Peru Balsam—*Myrosperum pereira, Myroxylon pereirae, Toluifera pereira*
Soybean—*Soja hispida*
Tolu Balsam—*Myroxylon balsamum*
Tonka Bean (*Tonquin Bean*)—*Baryosma tongo, Coumarouna odorata, Dipteryx odorata*

Fagaceae

Beechnut—*Fagus grandifolia, F. sylvatica*

Flacourtiaceae

Chaulmoogra—*Hypnocarpus kurzii, H. laurifolia, Taraktagenos kurzii, Oncoba echinata*

Geraniaceae

Geranium—*Pelargonium graveolens*

Grossulariaceae

Black Currant Seed—*Ribes nigrum*

Guttiferae

Calophyllum—*Calophyllum inophyllum*
Mangosteen (*Kokum Butter*)—*Garcinia mangostana*
St. John's Wort—*Hypericum perforatum*

Hamamelidaceae

Styrax (*Liquidamber* or *Storax*)—*Balsam styracis, Liquidamber orientalis, L. styraciflua*

Illiciaceae

Anise (*Star*)—*Illicium verum*

Iridaceae

Orris Root—*Iris florentina, I. pallida*
Saffron—*Crocus sativus*

Juglandaceae

Pecan—*Carya illinoinensis*
Walnut—*Juglans regia*

Lamiaceae

Basil (*Sweet*)—*Ocimum basilicum*
Calamint (*Catnip*)—*Calamintha clinopodium, C. officinalis, Nepeta cataria, Satureja calamintha*
Clary Sage—*Salvia sclarea*
Cornmint—*Mentha arvensis*
Hyssop—*Hyssopus officinalis*
Hyssop Decumbens—*Hyssopus officinalis* var. *decumbens*
Lavandin—*Lavandula fragrans, L. hortensis, L. hybrida*
Lavender—*Lavandula augustifolia, L. officinalis, L. vera*
Marjoram (*Spanish*)—*Thymus mastichina*
Marjoram (*Sweet*)—*Majorana hortensis, Origanum majorana*
Melissa (*Lemon Balm*)—*Melissa officinalis*
Monarda—*Monarda fistulosa*
Oregano—*Origanum vulgare*
Patchouli—*Pogostemon cablin, P. patchouli*
Pennyroyal—*Mentha pulegium*
Peppermint—*Mentha piperita*
Rosemary—*Rosmarinus coronarium, R. officinalis*
Sage—*Salvia officinalis*
Sage (*Spanish*)—*Salvia lavandulifolia*
Savory—*Calamintha hortensis, Satureja hortensis, S. montana*
Spearmint—*Mentha spicata, M. virdis*
Thyme—*Thymus aestivus, T. citriodora, T. ilerdensis, T. satureiodes, T. valentianus, T. vulgaris, T. vulgaris* var. *linalol, T. webbianus*

Lauraceae

Avocado—*Persea americana, P. gratissima*
Bay (*Sweet*)—*Laurus nobilis*
Bois de Rose (*Rosewood*)—*Aniba rosaeodora*
Camphor—*Cinnamomum camphora, Laurus camphora*

Cassia—*Cinnamomum aromaticum, C. cassia, Laurus cassia*
Cinnamon Bark and Leaf—*Cinnamomum verum, C. zeylanicum, Laurus cinnamomum*
Litsea Cubeba—*Litsea citrata, L. cubeba*
Massoia Bark—*Cryptocarya massoia*
Ravensara Anisata (*Havozo Bark*)—*Cinnamonum camphora, Ravensara anisata*
Ravensara Aromatica—*Cinnamonum camphora, Ravensara aromatica*
Sassafras—*Sassafras albidum*

Lecythidaceae

Brazil Nut—*Bertholletia excelsa*

Liliaceae

Aloe Vera—*Aloe barbadensis*

Linaceae

Flaxseed—*Linum usitatissimum*

Magnoliaceae

Champaca—*Michelia alba, M. champaca*

Malvaceae

Ambrette Seed—*Abelmoschus moschatus, Hibiscus abelmoschus*
Cottonseed—*Gossypium species*

Meliaceae

Neem—*Azadirachta indica*

Mimosaceae

Cassie—*Acacia farnesiana, Cassia ancienne*
Mimosa—*Acacia dealbata, A. decurrens*

Moraceae

Hops—*Humulus lupulus*

Moringaceae

Ben—*Moringa oleifera, M. pterygosperma*

Myristicaceae

Nutmeg—*Myristica aromata, M. fragrans, M. officinalis*

Myrtaceae

Allspice (*Pimento*)—*Pimenta dioica, P. officinalis*
Bay (*West Indian*)—*Myrcia acris, Pimenta acris, P. racemosa*
Cajeput—*Melaleuca cajuputi, M. leucadendron, M. minor*
Clove—*Eugenia aromatica, E. caryophyllata, E. caryophyllus, Syzygium aromaticum*
Eucalyptus—*Eucalyptus globulus*
Eucalyptus Citriodora—*Eucalyptus citriodora*
Eucalyptus Radiata—*Eucalyptus radiata*
Leptospermum (*New Zealand Tea Tree*)—*Leptospermum citratum, L. ericoides* (Kanuka), *L. scoparium* (Manuka), *L. petersonii*
Myrtle—*Myrtus communis*
Niaouli—*Melaleuca quinquenervia, M. viridiflora*
Tea Tree—*Melaleuca alternifolia, M. linariifolia, M. uncinata*

Oleaceae

Jasmine—*Jasminum officinale*
Olive—*Olea europaea*
Osmanthus—*Osmanthus fragrans*

Onagraceae

Evening Primrose—*Oenothera biennis*

Orchidaceae

Vanilla—*Vanilla fragrans, V. planifolia*

Passifloraceae

Passionflower—*Passiflora incarnata*

Pedaliaceae

Sesame—*Sesamum indicum*

Pinaceae

Cedarwood (*Atlas*)—*Cedrus atlantica*
Fir Balsam Needles—*Abies balsamea*
Fir Balsam Resin—*Abies balsamea, A. balsamifera, Pinus balsaamea*
Fir Needles—*Abies alba, A. grandis*
Larch—*Larix europaea*
Pine—*Pinus sylvestris*
Pine Nut—*Pinus edulis, P. pinea*

Spruce—*Picea mariana*
Spruce-Hemlock—*Tsuga canadensis*
Spruce-Sitka—*Picea sitchensis*
Terebinth—*Pinus maritima, P. palustris*

Piperaceae

Cubeb—*Cubeba officinalis, Piper cubeba*
Pepper (*Black*)—*Piper nigrum*

Poaceae

Citronella—*Andropogon nardus, Cymbopogon nardus*
Corn—*Zea mays*
Gingergrass—*Cymbopogon martinii* var. *sofia*
Lemongrass—*Cymbopogon citratus, C. flexosus*
Palmarosa—*Andronpogon martinii, Cymbopogon martinii* var. *motia*
Rice Bran—*Oryza sativa*
Vetiver—*Andropogon muricatus, Vetiveria zizanoides*
Wheat Germ—*Triticum vulgare*

Protoceae

Macadamia Nut—*Macadamia integrifolia*

Rosaceae

Almond (*Sweet*)—*Prunus amygdalus, P. dulcis*
Apricot Kernel—*Armeniaca vulgaris, Prunus armeniaca*
Rose—*Rosa centifolia, R. damascena*
Rose Hip Seed—*Rosa rubiginosa*

Rubiaceae

Coffee—*Coffea arabica*
Gardenia—*Gardenia grandiflora*

Rutaceae

Amyris—*Amyris balsamifera, Schimmelia oleifera*
Bergamot—*Citrus bergamia*
Grapefruit—*Citrus paradisi, C. racemosa*
Lemon—*Citrus limon*
Lime—*Citrus aurantiifolia, C. limetta*
Mandarin—*Citrus madurensis, C. nobilis, C. reticulata*
Neroli—*Citrus aurantium*
Orange (*Bitter*)—*Citrus aurantium*
Orange (*Sweet*)—*Citrus sinensis*

Petitgrain—*Citrus bigaradia*
Rue—*Ruta graveolens*
Tangelo—*Citrus tangelo*
Tangerine—*Citrus reticulata*
Temple Orange—*Citrus reticulata*
Zanthoxylum—*Zanthoxylum alatum, Z. americanum, Z. rhesta*

Santalaceae

Sandalwood—*Santalum album*

Sapotaceae

Shea Butter—*Butyrosperum parkii*

Simmondsaceae

Jojoba—*Simmondsia chinensis*

Solanaceae

Tobacco Leaf—*Nicotiana tabacum*

Sterculiaceae

Cocoa Butter—*Theobroma cacao*

Styracaceae

Benzoin—*Styrax benzoin, S. tonkinensis*

Theaceae

Camellia—*Camellia japonica*

Tiliaceae

Linden Blossom—*Tilia europaea, T. vulgaris*

Valerianaceae

Spikenard—*Nardostachys jatamansi*
Valerian—*Valeriana officinalis*

Verbenaceae

Lantana—*Lantana camara*
Lemon Verbena—*Aloysia citriodora, A. triphylla, Lippia citriodora, L. triphylla, Verbena triphylla*

Violaceae

Violet—*Viola odorata*

Vitaceae
Grapeseed—*Vitis vinifera*

Zingiberaceae

Cardamom—*Elettaria cardamomum*
Galangal—*Alpinia officinarum, Languas officinarum*
Ginger—*Zingiber officinale*
Turmeric—*Amomoum curcuma, Curcuma domestica, C. longa*

Zygophyllaceae

Guaiacwood—*Bulnesia sarmienti, Guaiacum officinale*

Glossary

ABORTIFACIENT: Abortion. Induces childbirth or premature labor.

AEROPHAGY: A buildup of air in the body that is relieved through burping or flatulence.

ALTERATIVE: Produces a gradual improvement on the nutritional state of the body.

ANALGESIC: Relieves or reduces pain.

ANAPHRODISIAC: Reduces sexual desire.

ANESTHETIC: Numbs the nerves and causes a loss of sensation.

ANTHELMINTIC: Expels or kills intestinal worms.

ANTIBACTERIAL: Prevents the growth of and kills bacteria.

ANTIDEPRESSANT: Alleviates or prevents depression.

ANTIDIARRHOEIC: Relieves diarrhea.

ANTIDOTE: A remedy to counteract a poison.

ANTIEMETIC: Counteracts nausea and stops vomiting.

ANTIFUNGAL: Kills fungal infections.

ANTIGALACTAGOGUE: Lessens the production of milk secretion of nursing mothers.

ANTI-INFLAMMATORY: Reduces inflammation.

ANTILITHIC: Prevents formation of stones or calculus.

ANTINEURALGIC: Stops nerve pain.

ANTIPHLOGISTIC: Counteracts, reduces, or prevents inflammation.

ANTIPRURITIC: Relieves or prevents itching.

ANTIPUTRID: Stops putrefaction.

ANTISCLEROTIC: Removes deposits from circulatory vessels and the body.

ANTISCORBUTIC: Preventative for scurvy.

ANTISEPTIC: Inhibits the growth of and kills bacteria.

ANTISPASMODIC: Relieves or prevents spasms, cramps, and convulsions.

ANTISUDORIFIC: Stops perspiration.

ANTITOXIC: Counteracts poisons.

ANTITUSSIVE: Relieves coughs.

ANTIVIRAL: Weakens and kills viruses.

APERIENT: A gentle purgative of the bowels.

APERITIF: An alcoholic drink taken to stimulate the appetite before a meal.

APERITIVE: Stimulates the appetite.

APHRODISIAC: Arouses sexual desires.

ASTRINGENT: Contracts tissue and reduces secretions.

BALSAMIC: Softens phlegm.

BRONCHODILATOR: Dilates the spastic bronchial tube.

CALMATIVE: Mild sedative or tranquilizer.

CARDIAC: Stimulates or affects the heart.

CARDIOTONIC: Tones the heart muscle.

CARMINATIVE: Expels gas from the intestines.

CAUSTIC: Can damage skin tissue through chemical action.

CEPHALIC: Problems relating to the head.

CHOLAGOGUE: Increases the flow of bile.

CHOLERETIC: Stimulates the production of bile.

CICATRIZANT: Helps the formation of scar tissue; healing.

COAGULANT: Clots the blood.

CORDIAL: Stimulant and tonic.

COUNTER-IRRITANT: An irritant used to counteract irritation or inflammation in another part of the body.

CYTOPHYLACTIC: Protects the cells of the organism.

DECONGESTANT: Relieves congestion.

DEMULCENT: Soothes irritated tissue, particularly mucous membranes.

DEODORANT: Deodorizer. Eliminates offensive odors.

DEPURATIVE: Cleanses and purifies the blood and internal organs.

DETERSIVE: Detergent. Cleanses wounds and sores, and promotes the formation of scar tissue.

DIAPHORETIC: Causes perspiration.

DIGESTIVE: Promotes and aids digestion.

DISINFECTANT: Kills infections and disease-producing microorganisms.

DIURETIC: Increases the secretion and elimination of urine.

EMETIC: Induces vomiting.

EMMENAGOGUE: Promotes and regulates menstruation.

EMOLLIENT: Softens the skin, and soothes inflamed and irritated tissues.

ESTROGENIC: Similar to estrogen.

EUPHORIANT: Brings on an exaggerated sense of physical and emotional well-being.

EXPECTORANT: Promotes the discharge of mucous from the lungs and bronchial tubes.

FEBRIFUGE: Reduces or prevents fevers.

FIXATIVE: Holds the scent of a fragrance.

GALACTAGOGUE: Promotes or increases the secretion of milk in nursing mothers.

GERMICIDE: Kills germs.

HALLUCINOGEN: Induces hallucinations—an imagined or false sense of perception.

HEMOSTATIC: Stops hemorrhaging.

HEPATIC: Acts on the liver.

HYPERTENSOR: Raises the blood pressure.

HYPNOTIC: Induces sleep.

HYPOTENSOR: Lowers the blood pressure.

INSECT REPELLENT: Repels insects.

INSECTICIDE: Kills insects.

LARVICIDE: Kills the larvae of insects.

LAXATIVE: Promotes the evacuation of the bowels; a mild purgative.

NERVINE: Calming and soothing to the nervous system.

PARASITICIDE: Kills parasites, especially those living on or in the skin.

PECTORAL: Having an effect on the respiratory system.

PURGATIVE: Promotes a vigorous evacuation of the bowels.

REFRIGERANT: Cools and lowers the body temperature.

REGENERATOR: Promotes new growth or repair of structures or tissues lost by disease or injury.

REJUVENATOR: To make young again and bring back the youthful appearance.

RELAXANT: Lessens or reduces tension, and produces relaxation.

RESOLVENT: Disperses swellings.

RESTORATIVE: Restores consciousness and/or normal physiological activity.

RUBEFACIENT: A local irritant that reddens the skin.

SEDATIVE: Calms anxiety and promotes drowsiness.

STIMULANT: Excites or quickens an activity in the body.

STOMACHIC: Strengthens, stimulates, and tones the stomach.

SUDORIFIC: Promotes or increases perspiration.

TONIC: Strengthens and invigorates the entire body or specific organs.

TRANQUILIZER: Calms the nerves and brings on a state of peacefulness without inducing sleep.

VASOCONSTRICTOR: Constricts the blood vessels, which raises the blood pressure.

VASODILATOR: Dilates the blood vessels.

VERMIFUGE: Expels intestinal worms.

VULNERARY: Heals wounds and sores by external application.

Bibliography

Aihara, Herman. *Basic Macrobiotics*. Japan Publications, 1985.

Angier, Bradford. *Field Guide to Medicinal Wild Plants*. Stackpole Books, 1978.

Arasaki, Seiban and Arasaki, Teruko. *Vegetables from the Sea*. Japan Publications.

Ayensu, Edward S. *Our Green and Living World*. Cambridge University Press, 1984.

Bianchini, Francesco. *Health Plants of the World*. Newsweek Books, 1975.

Bown, Deni. *Encyclopedia of Herbs & Their Uses*. Dorling Kindersley, 1995.

Bremness, Lesley. *The Complete Book of Herbs*. Viking Penguin, 1988.

Bremness, Lesley. *Herbs*. Dorling Kindersley, 1994.

Carper, Jean. *The Food Pharmacy*. Bantam Books, 1988.

Carroll, Anstice. *The Health Food Dictionary*. Weathervane Books.

Cavendish, Marshall. *Illustrated Book of Trees and Forests of the World*. Marshall Cavendish, 1990.

Cunningham, Donna. *Flower Remedies Handbook: Emotional Healing & Growth with Bach & Other Flower Essences*. Sterling Publishing Company, 1992.

Dorfler, Dr. Hans-Peter, and Roselt, Prof. Gerhard. *The Dictionary of Healing Plants*. Blandford Press, London, 1989.

Duff, Gail. *A Book of Herbs and Spices*. Salem House Pub., 1987.

Duke, James A. *Handbook of Medicinal Plants*. CRC Press, 1985.

Duke, James A. *Handbook of NorthEastern Indian Medicinal Plants*. Quarterman Pub., 1986.

Duke, James A. *Handbook of Nuts*. CRC Press, 1989.

Erasmus, Udo. *Fats and Oils*. Alive, 1986.

Erdmann, Robert and Meirion, Jones. *Fats, Health and Nutrition*. Thorsons Publishing Group, 1990.

Farrell, Kenneth T. *Spices, Condiments and Seasonings*. Avi Publishing, 1985.

Fischer-Rizzi, Susanne. *Complete Aromatherapy Handbook: Essential Oils for Radiant Health*. Sterling Publishing Company, 1990.

Foster, Steven and Duke, James A. *A Field Guide to Medicinal Plants*. Houghton Mifflin, 1990.

Franchomme, Pierre and Pénoël, Daniel. *L'Aromathérapie Exactement*. Roger Jollois (Editeur), 1995.

Genders, Roy. *Cosmetics from the Earth*. Alfred van der Mark Editions, 1986.

Graham, Judy. *Evening Primrose Oil*. Thorsons Publishers Inc., 1984.

Griffith, Mark. *Index of Garden Plants*. Timber Press, 1992.

Groom, Nigel. *The Perfume Handbook*. Chapman and Hall, 1992.

Gurudas. *Flower Essences and Vibrational Healing*. Brotherhood of Life, 1983.

Hampton, Aubrey. *Natural Organic Hair and Skin Care*. Organica Press, 1987.

Harrison, S.G. *The Oxford Book of Food Plants*. Oxford University Press, 1969.

Huang, Kee Chang. *The Pharmacology of Chinese Herbs*. CRC Press, 1993.

Hurley, Judith Benn. *The Good Herb*. William Morrow Company, 1995.

Hutchens, Alma. *Indian Herbalogy of North America*. Merco, 1973.

Keville, Kathi. *The Illustrated Herb Encyclopedia*. Mallard Press, 1991.

Kushi, Michio. *Macrobiotic Home Remedies*. Japan Publications, 1985.

Lavabre, Marcel. *Aromatherapy Workbook*. Healing Arts Press, 1990.

Lawless, Julia. *The Encyclopedia of Essential Oils*. Element Books, 1992.

Leung, Albert Y. *Chinese Herbal Remedies*. Phaidon Universe, 1984.

Leung, Albert Y. *Encyclopedia of Common Natural Ingredients*. John Wiley & Sons, 1980.

Levy, Juliette de Bairacli. *Common Herbs for Natural Health*. Schocken Books, 1971.

Lowenfield, Claire, and Back, Philippa. *The Complete Book of Herbs and Spices*. G.P. Putnams, 1974.

Lust, John. *The Herb Book*. Bantam Books, 1974.

Mabberley, D.J. *The Plant Book*. Cambridge University Press, 1987.

Mairesse, Michelle. *Health Secrets of Medicinal Herbs*. Arco Pub., 1981.

Martin, Laura C. *Wildflower Folklore*. East Woods Press, 1984.

Menninger, Edwin A. *Edible Nuts of the World*. Horticulture Books, 1977.

Morton, Julia F. *Fruits of Warm Climates*. Julia F. Morton, 1987.

National Academy Press. *Neem, A Tree for Solving Global Problems*. National Academy Press, 1992.

Ody, Penelope. *The Complete Medicinal Herbal*. Dorling Kindersly, 1993.

Price, Shirley. *Aromatherapy for Common Ailments*. Gaia Books Limited, 1991.

Price, Shirley. *Aromatherapy Workbook*. Thorsons, 1993.

Reader's Digest. *Magic and Medicine of Plants*. Reader's Digest, 1986.

Rosengarten, Frederic, Jr. *The Book of Spices*. Pyramid Books, 1973.

Rosengarten, Frederic, Jr. *The Book of Edible Nuts*. Walker and Company, 1984.

Ryman, Daniele. *The Complete Guide to Plants and Flower Essences for Health and Beauty*. Bantam Books, 1993.

Sadler, Julie. *Aromatherapy: Family Matters*. Sterling Publishing Company, 1991.

Sanecki, Kay N. *The Complete Book of Herbs*. Macmillan, 1974.

Santillo, Humbart. *Natural Healing with Herbs*. Hohn Press, 1984.

Schiller, Carol and Schiller, David. *500 Formulas for Aromatherapy*. Sterling Publishing Company, 1994.

Schiller, Carol and Schiller, David. *Aromatherapy for Mind and Body*. Sterling Publishing Company, 1996.

Sellar, Wanda. *The Directory of Essential Oils*. C.W. Daniel Company Limited 1992.

Thomson, William A.R., MD. *Medicines from the Earth*. McGraw Hill, 1978.

Tierra, Michael. *The Way of Herbs*. Unity Press, 1980.

Tierra, Michael. *Planetary Herbology*. Lotus Press, 1988.

Tisserand, Robert. *The Art of Aromatherapy*. Healing Arts Press, 1975.

Toussaint-Samat, Maguelonne. *History of Food*. Blackwell Publishers, 1992.

Valnet, Jean. *Organic Garden Medicine*. Erbonia Books, 1975.

Valnet, Jean. *The Practice of Aromatherapy.* Destiny Books, 1982.

Weiner, Michael A. *The People's Herbal.* Putnam Publishing, 1984.

Weiss, Gaea and Shandor. *Growing and Using the Healing Herbs.* Rodale Press, 1985.

Westland, Pamela. *The Encyclopedia of Spices.* Chartwell Books, 1979.

Wildwood, Chrissie. *Erotic Aromatherapy: Essential Oils for Lovers.* Sterling Publishing Company, 1994.

Worwood, Valerie Ann. *The Complete Book of Essential Oils and Aromatherapy.* New World Library, 1991.

Index

About the Authors

Carol Schiller and David Schiller have been instructing aromatherapy classes for colleges as well as other educational organizations since 1989, and formulating essential oil blends since 1986. They are the authors of *500 Formulas for Aromatherapy* (Sterling), *Aromatherapy for Mind & Body* (Sterling), and numerous magazine articles.

Carol Schiller is also a certified hypnotherapist and graphologist, and instructs classes on these subjects as well.

Jeffrey Schiller, the illustrator of this book, is the founder and president of the International Aromatherapy and Herb Association (IAHA), and editor of *Making Scents,* the association's newsletter.